NEUROSCIENCE RESE

MOTOR IMAGERY

EMERGING PRACTICES, ROLE IN PHYSICAL THERAPY AND CLINICAL IMPLICATIONS

NEUROSCIENCE RESEARCH PROGRESS

Additional books in this series can be found on Nova's website
under the Series tab.

Additional e-books in this series can be found on Nova's website
under the e-book tab.

NEUROSCIENCE RESEARCH PROGRESS

MOTOR IMAGERY

EMERGING PRACTICES, ROLE IN PHYSICAL THERAPY AND CLINICAL IMPLICATIONS

BRANDON M. GARCIA
EDITOR

New York

Library of Congress Cataloging-in-Publication Data

ISBN: 978-1-63483-125-3
Library of Congress Control Number: 2015942065

Published by Nova Science Publishers, Inc. † New York

Contents

Preface

Motor imagery, the mental rehearsal of a motor act without overt movement, has been shown to improve motor performance in healthy subjects. It is well known that motor imagery has the potential to promote greater insight to the development of action planning, because of that, it is now considered a fundamental topic of study in the field of motor behavior. This book addresses emerging practices, the role of motor imagery in physical therapy, and clinical implications of motor imagery as well.

Chapter 1 – Motor imagery, the mental rehearsal of a motor act without overt movement, has been shown to improve motor performance in healthy subjects. It also aids in the recovery of motor function following stroke effects of motor imagery have shown that corticospinal excitability during motor imagery may result from an increase in the MEP amplitude, as measured by transcranial magnetic stimulation (TMS). However, the H-reflex, T-wave, and F-wave measurements as indices of the excitability of spinal neural function during motor imagery were not obtained in these studies. If motor imagery is used as part of a patient's rehabilitation, it has the potential to increase both motor cortical function and spinal neural function. In turn, improved spinal neural function can result in improved muscle function. Our final goal of motor imagery research is to identify the best method to improve the excitability of spinal neural function in the clinical setting.

We would like to introduce our study on motor imagery. At first, we introduce the study entitled "Excitability of Spinal Neural Function during Several Motor Imagery Tasks involving Isometric Opponens Pollicis Activity." Motor imagery under the "with sensor" and "without sensor" conditions at approximately 50% MVC of the opponens pollicis without overt motor output increased the excitability of spinal neural output to the thenar muscles. Because the relative data for the persistence and F/M amplitude ratio during motor imagery under the "with sensor" condition were higher than those during that under the "without sensor" condition, the movement preparation for a motor imagery task involving 50% MVC of the opponens pollicis is extremely important.

Next, we introduce the study entitled "Excitability of Spinal Neural Function by Motor Imagery with Isometric Opponens Pollicis Activity: Influence of Vision during Motor Imagery." Motor imagery while maintaining 50% MVC of the opponens pollicis muscle without overt motor output with a subject's eyes open or closed increased the excitability of spinal neural output to the subject's thenar muscles. There was no significant difference in the excitability of spinal neural function by motor imagery under these conditions. The subjective evaluations illustrated that motor imagery with the subject's eyes open or closed had no effect on motor imagery.

Finally, we introduce the study "Excitability of Spinal Neural Function during Motor Imagery in Parkinson's disease. "Motor imagery under both the "with sensor" and "without sensor" conditions at approximately 50% MVC of the opponens pollicis without overt motor output increased the excitability of spinal neural output to the thenar muscles in 10 patients with Parkinson's disease. Because persistence and the F/M amplitude ratio during motor imagery under the "with sensor" condition were significantly higher compared with those at rest, movement preparation for a motor imagery task involving 50% MVC of the opponens pollicis is extremely important.

Chapter 2 – Developmental Coordination Disorder (DCD) is a disorder that defines children with problems in their motor coordination development despite their intelligence levels and impacts about 2-7% of school-age children. While the degree of motor impairment varies, common symptoms of the disorder include marked delays in achieving motor milestones and clumsiness, normally associated with poor balance, coordination, and handwriting skills. These difficulties associated with motor learning and control may last well into adolescence and adulthood. In this chapter, I will provide a description of how children with DCD are said to have difficulties with motor imagery (MI), i.e., the ability to mentally representing motor behavior, planning and generating an accurate visuospatial representation of an intended action, and coupling sensory information with appropriate motor actions. The neurocognitive perspective states that this problem results from an underlying deficit in generating and/or monitoring internal models of action, termed the internal modeling deficit (IMD) hypothesis. This hypothesis has been largely accepted as one of the likely causes of the motor skill difficulties presented in DCD. The understanding of the IMD hypothesis and how children with DCD use motor imagery offers practical applications for the understanding of screening, diagnostic, and rehabilitation protocols in physical therapy. Here, I will also explore such clinical implications and provide suggestions and strategies for rehabilitation in these children.

Chapter 3 – Contemporary research findings indicate that in older persons (typically 64 > years) there are functional decrements in the ability to mentally represent and effectively plan motor actions. That is, many older persons do not effectively simulate (via mental imagery) prior actions resulting in intentions that are significantly different from movement execution. For example, our work and others have reported that, compared to younger adults, older persons typically show greater over- or underestimation of abilities, such as when reaching and stepping. Such incorrections may, especially with the elderly, lead to loss of postural control (balance) and a higher risk of falling. This chapter: (1) highlights research findings on mental representation and motor imagery in the elderly, (2) describes the effectiveness and potential of motor imagery training in general, (3) addresses the implications for improving movement efficiency and lowering the risk of movement-related injury, and finally, (4) provides guidelines / strategies for motor imagery practice in the context of reach planning.

Chapter 4 – A brain-computer interface (BCI) analyzes brain activity in real-time to convey information or control an external device. BCI systems often consist of a biosignal amplifier for EEG data acquisition, parameter estimation, and classification to make decisions in real-time. Many BCIs are controlled via motor imagery (through imagined movements), which modulates the EEG in certain frequency bands and regions. Motor imagery based BCIs are used for various applications like cursor control, robotic and avatar control, stroke rehabilitation, cognitive assessment, training, and communication. This article presents key scientific experiments and applications, including some of the newest results.

Chapter 5 – Motor imagery is an active cognitive strategy requiring the internal reproduction of a specific action without any overt motor output. Mental practice is a method by which the internal reproduction of a given motor act - the motor imagery - is extensively repeated. This method is defined as a mental rehearsal of kinesthetic and/or visual properties of movements. Actually, many studies showed that mental practice improves the functional performance in neurologic and orthopedic injuries associated with change in neural activation related to motor control. Usually this approach increases activation in motor areas related to planning and preparation and decreases activation in primary motor areas. This intervention can be used in physical therapy to improve motor relearning in individuals with different motor impairments and physical functional disabilities. However, the definition of parameters is necessary to guide the application of this method in clinical practice. This chapter describes aspects related to the use of motor imagery in clinical practice, including: a) main indications in different injury stages, b) neurophysiologic aspects improving motor recovery in individuals with motor impairments, c) clinical parameters in physical therapy, including the assessment process, session's characteristics and follow-up, and d) clinical applicability. Many variables, such as the nature of motor tasks, practice intensity, duration, learning stages, as well as individual aspects, need to be considered to guide clinical practice. The knowledge of these variables helps to apply this approach in clinical contexts.

In: Motor Imagery
Editor: Brandon M. Garcia

ISBN: 978-1-63483-125-3

Chapter 1

Spinal Neural Function during Motor Imagery

Toshiaki Suzuki[1,2], Yoshibumi Bunno[1,2], Makiko Tani[1,2], Chieko Onigata[2], Hirohisa Yoneda[1,2], Marina Todo[1], Sayuri Uragami[2], Ikuro Wakayama[1] and Sohei Yoshida[1]

[1]Graduate School of Health Sciences, Graduate School of Kansai University of Health Sciences, Japan

[2]Clinical Physical Therapy Laboratory, Faculty of Health Sciences, Kansai University of Health Sciences, Japan

Abstract

Motor imagery, the mental rehearsal of a motor act without overt movement, has been shown to improve motor performance in healthy subjects (Pascual-Leone et al., 1995). It also aids in the recovery of motor function following stroke (Ryding, Decety, Sjoholm, Stenberg, & Ingvar, 1993; Stevens & Stoykov, 2003). The effects of motor imagery have shown that corticospinal excitability during motor imagery may result from an increase in the MEP amplitude, as measured by transcranial magnetic stimulation (TMS) (Hashimoto & Rothwell, 1999; Li, Latash, & Zatsiorsky, 2004). However, the H-reflex, T-wave, and F-wave measurements as indices of the excitability of spinal neural function during motor imagery were not obtained in these studies (Hale et al, 2003; Jeannerod, 1995; Kasai et al., 1997; Oishi et al, 1994). If motor imagery is used as part of a patient's rehabilitation, it has the potential to increase both motor cortical function and spinal neural function. In turn, improved spinal neural function can result in improved muscle function. Our final goal of motor imagery research is to identify the best method to improve the excitability of spinal neural function in the clinical setting.

We would like to introduce our study on motor imagery. At first, we introduce the study entitled "Excitability of Spinal Neural Function during Several Motor Imagery Tasks involving Isometric Opponens Pollicis Activity (Suzuki et al., 2013)." Motor imagery under the "with sensor" and "without sensor" conditions at approximately 50% MVC of the opponens pollicis without overt motor output increased the excitability of spinal neural output to the thenar muscles. Because the relative data for the persistence and F/M amplitude ratio during motor imagery under the "with sensor" condition were higher than those during that under the "without sensor" condition, the movement preparation for a motor imagery task involving 50% MVC of the opponens pollicis is extremely important.

Next, we introduce the study entitled "Excitability of Spinal Neural Function by Motor Imagery with Isometric Opponens Pollicis Activity: Influence of Vision during Motor Imagery (Suzuki et al., 2014)." Motor imagery while maintaining 50% MVC of the opponens pollicis muscle without overt motor output with a subject's eyes open or closed increased the excitability of spinal neural output to the subject's thenar muscles. There was no significant difference in the excitability of spinal neural function by motor imagery under these conditions. The subjective evaluations illustrated that motor imagery with the subject's eyes open or closed had no effect on motor imagery.

Finally, we introduce the study "Excitability of Spinal Neural Function during Motor Imagery in Parkinson's disease (Suzuki et al., 2014)."Motor imagery under both the "with sensor" and "without sensor" conditions at approximately 50% MVC of the opponens pollicis without overt motor output increased the excitability of spinal neural output to the thenar muscles in 10 patients with Parkinson's disease. Because persistence and the F/M amplitude ratio during motor imagery under the "with sensor" condition were significantly higher compared with those at rest, movement preparation for a motor imagery task involving 50% MVC of the opponens pollicis is extremely important.

1. Introduction

Motor imagery, the mental rehearsal of a motor act without overt movement, has been shown to improve motor performance in healthy subjects (Pascual-Leone et al., 1995). It also aids in the recovery of motor function following stroke (Ryding, Decety, Sjoholm, Stenberg, & Ingvar, 1993; Stevens & Stoykov, 2003). The effects of motor imagery have been discussed in many neurophysiological studies using motor-evoked potentials (MEPs), the Hoffman reflex (H-reflex), the T-wave, and the F-wave. Results have shown that corticospinal excitability during motor imagery may result from an increase in the MEP amplitude, as measured by transcranial magnetic stimulation (TMS) (Hashimoto & Rothwell, 1999; Li, Latash, & Zatsiorsky, 2004). However, the H-reflex, T-wave, and F-wave measurements as indices of the excitability of spinal neural function during motor imagery were not obtained in these studies (Hale et al, 2003; Jeannerod, 1995; Kasai et al., 1997; Oishi et al, 1994). Motor imagery may be more precisely defined as imagery that produces spatial and temporal modulation of motor cortical function that mirrors the modulation observed during the actual performance of a task without activation of spinal neural function. If motor imagery is used as part of a patient's rehabilitation, it has the potential to increase both motor cortical function and spinal neural function. In turn, improved spinal neural function can result in improved muscle function. Our final goal of motor imagery research is to identify the best method to improve the excitability of spinal neural function in the clinical setting.

We would like to introduce our study on motor imagery. However, first, we introduce the study entitled "Excitability of Spinal Neural Function during Several Motor Imagery Tasks involving Isometric Opponens Pollicis Activity (Suzuki et al., 2013)." This research founded the best method of motor imagery in healthy persons. Next, we introduce the study entitled "Excitability of Spinal Neural Function by Motor Imagery with Isometric Opponens Pollicis Activity: Influence of Vision during Motor Imagery (Suzuki et al., 2014)." This study had evaluated the influence of vision on motor imagery in healthy subjects. Finally, we introduce the study "Excitability of Spinal Neural Function during Motor Imagery in Parkinson's disease (Suzuki et al., 2014)."

2. Excitability of Spinal Neural Function during Several Motor Imagery Tasks Involving Isometric Opponens Pollicis Activity (Suzuki et al., 2013)

2.1. Purpose

In this study, subjects learned 50% maximal voluntary contraction (MVC) through isometric contraction of the opponens pollicis muscle by holding a pinch meter with a sensor between the thumb and index finger. Next, the subjects were asked to imagine the same contraction under two conditions: holding the sensor of pinch meter between the thumb and index finger ("with sensor"; holding condition) and not holding the sensor of pinch meter (without sensor"; resting condition). We aimed to determine whether mental simulation without the actual muscle contraction associated with the actual motion of holding the pinch meter and sensor can increase the excitability of spinal neural function.

During these motor imagery conditions, we tested the F-wave of the left thenar muscles after stimulating the left median nerve at the wrist. The F-wave resulted from the backfiring of the α-motoneurons after antidromic invasion of the propagated impulse across the axon hillock (Kimura, 1974). Its occurrence reflects excitability changes in the spinal motoneurons, as reported in patients with spasticity (Odusote & Eisen, 1979) and in healthy subjects with isometric contraction (Suzuki, Fujiwara, & Takeda, 1993).

2.2. Materials and Methods

2.2.1. Subjects

In total, 11 healthy volunteers (8 males and 3 females; mean age, 34 years) participated in the study. Written informed consent was obtained from all subjects. This study was approved by the Research Ethics Committee of Kansai University of Health Sciences. The experiments were conducted in accordance with the Declaration of Helsinki. There are no conflicts of interest associated with this study.

2.2.2. F-wave during Motor Imagery (Figure 1)

Subjects were positioned comfortably in a supine position with external rotation of both shoulder joints. The skin was prepared with abrasive gel to maintain the impedance below 5 KΩ. A Viking Quest electromyography machine (Natus Medical Inc., CA, USA) was used to record the F-waves. We tested the F-waves of the left thenar muscles with a pair of round disks attached (with collodion) to the skin over the belly and the bone of the metacarpophalangeal joint of the thumb after stimulating the left median nerve at the wrist at rest and under touch and motor imagery conditions. The stimulating electrodes comprised a cathode placed over the left median nerve at 3 cm proximal to the palmar crease of the wrist joint and an anode placed 2 cm further proximally. The maximal stimulus was determined by delivering 0.2-ms square-wave pulses of increasing intensity to elicit the largest compound muscle action potentials. Supramaximal shocks (adjusted up to a value of 20% higher than the maximal stimulus) were delivered at 0.5 Hz for the acquisition of F-waves. The bandwidth filter ranged from 2 Hz to 3 kHz.

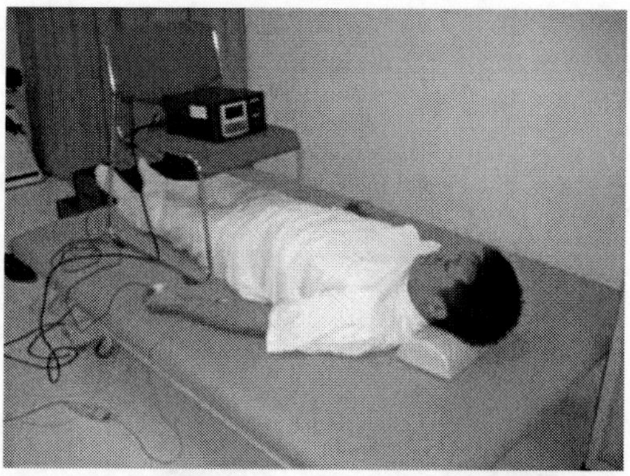

Figure 1. Test conditions.

In the resting condition, we tested the F-wave during relaxation. In the holding condition, the subject held the pinch meter and sensor between the thumb and index finger. For the motor imagery condition, subjects first learned 50% MVC through isometric contraction of the opponens pollicis muscle by holding the pinch meter. Next, the subjects were asked to imagine the contraction while holding the pinch meter and sensor between the thumb and index finger (motor imagery under the "with sensor" condition) on one day and while not holding the sensor on another day (motor imagery under the "without sensor" condition).

2.2.3. Data Analysis

The F-waves from 30 trials were analyzed with respect to persistence, the F/M amplitude ratio, and latency. Persistence was defined by the number of measurable F-wave responses divided by 30 trials of supramaximal stimulation. The F/M amplitude ratio was defined as the mean amplitude of all responses divided by the amplitude of the M-wave. Latency was defined as the mean latency from the time of stimulation to the onset of a measurable F-wave. Dunnett's test was used to compare results between the resting condition and the other two conditions. A paired *t*-test was used to compare F-wave results during motor imagery under the "with sensor" and "without sensor" conditions.

2.3. Results

2.3.1. F-Wave Results during Motor Imagery under the "with Sensor" Condition

Persistence during the holding condition and during motor imagery under the "with sensor" condition was significantly better than that observed at rest (Dunnett's test: *$p < 0.01$) (Figure 2).

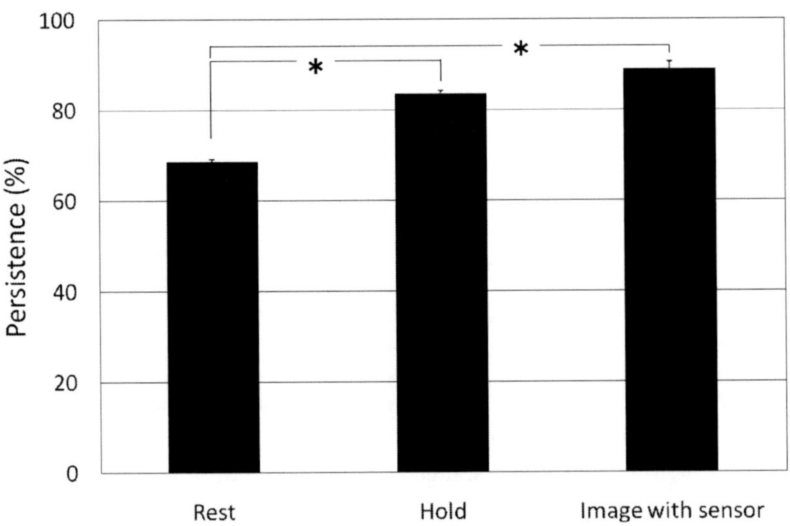

Figure 2. Persistence during resting, holding, and motor imagery under the "with sensor" condition. Persistence during the holding condition and during motor imagery under the "with sensor" condition was significantly better than that during the resting condition (Dunnett's test: *$p < 0.01$).

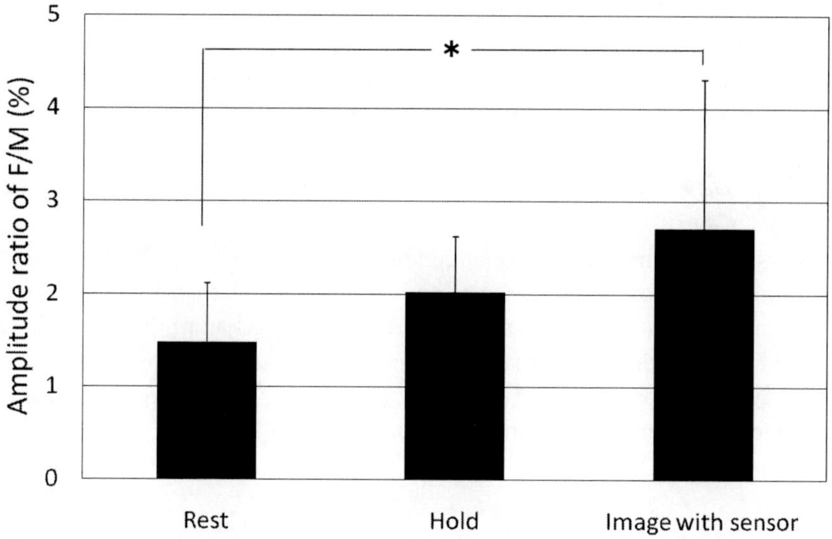

Figure 3. The F/M amplitude ratio during resting, holding, and motor imagery under the "with sensor" condition. The F/M amplitude ratio during motor imagery under the "with sensor" condition was significantly greater than that during the resting condition (Dunnett's test: $*p < 0.01$).

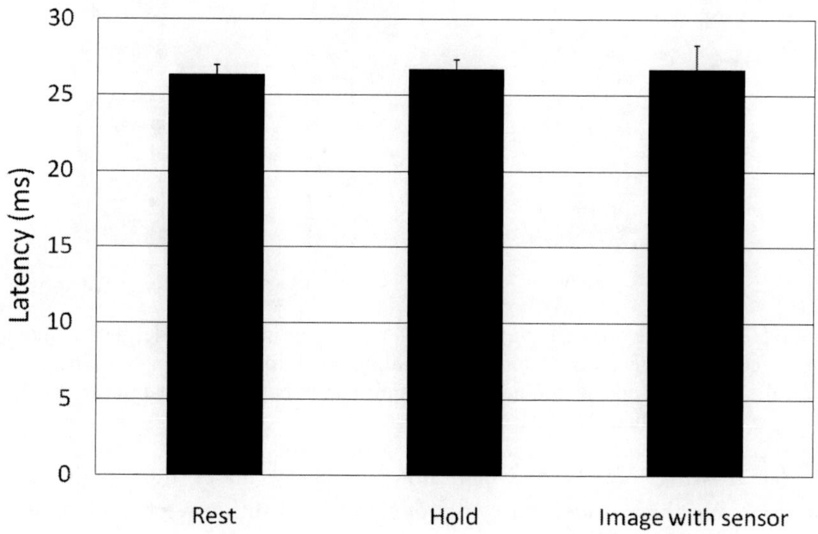

Figure 4. Latency during resting, holding, and motor imagery under the "with sensor" condition. There were no significant differences in latency among the three conditions.

In addition, the F/M amplitude ratio during motor imagery under the "with sensor" condition was significantly greater than that observed at rest (Dunnett's test: *p < 0.01) (Figure 3). There were no significant differences in latency among the three conditions (Figure 4).

2.3.2. F-wave Results during Motor Imagery under the "without Sensor" Condition

Persistence during the holding condition and during motor imagery under the "without sensor" condition was significantly better than that observed at rest (Dunnett's test: *p < 0.01) (Figure 5), and the F/M amplitude ratio during the holding condition and during motor imagery under the same condition was slightly greater than that observed at rest (Figure 6). There were no significant differences in latency among the three conditions (Figure 7).

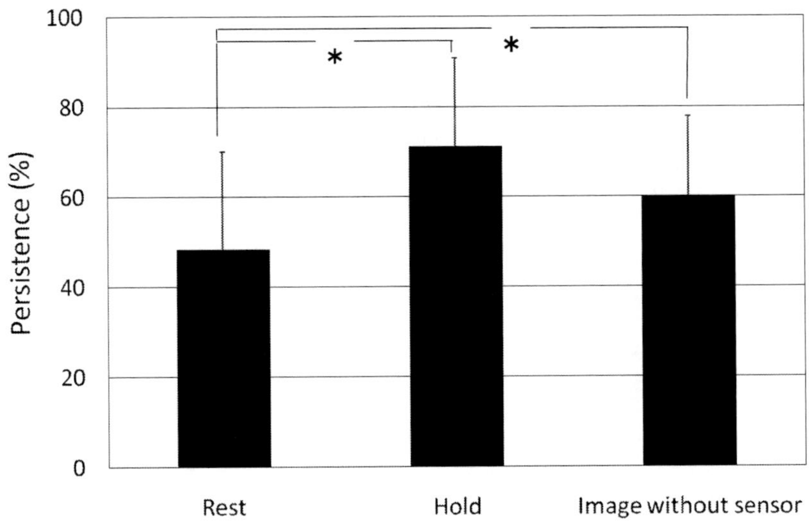

Figure 5. Persistence during resting, holding, and motor imagery under the "without sensor" condition. Persistence during the holding condition and during motor imagery under the "without sensor" condition was significantly better than that during the resting condition (Dunnett's test: *p < 0.01).

The F-wave results between motor imagery under the "with sensor" condition and those under the "without sensor" condition were compared. The relative persistence and F/M amplitude ratio during motor imagery under the "with sensor" condition were higher than those during motor imagery under the "without sensor" condition (Figures 8 and 9). In particular, the relative data for the F/M amplitude ratio during motor imagery under the "with sensor" condition was significantly higher than that during motor imagery under the "without sensor" condition (paired t-test: *$p < 0.05$) (Figure 9).

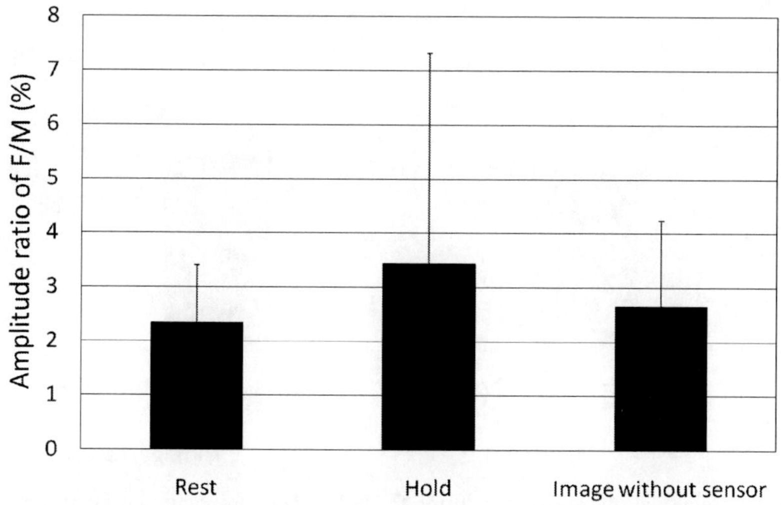

Figure 6. The F/M amplitude ratio during resting, holding, and motor imagery under the "without sensor" condition. The F/M amplitude ratio during the holding condition and during motor imagery under the "without sensor" condition was likely to increase compared with that during the resting condition.

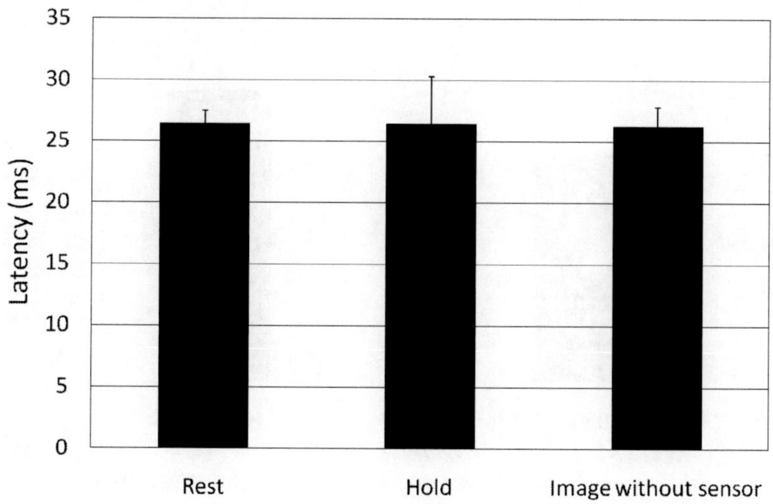

Figure 7. Latency during resting, holding, and motor imagery under the "without sensor" condition. There were no significant differences in latency among the three conditions.

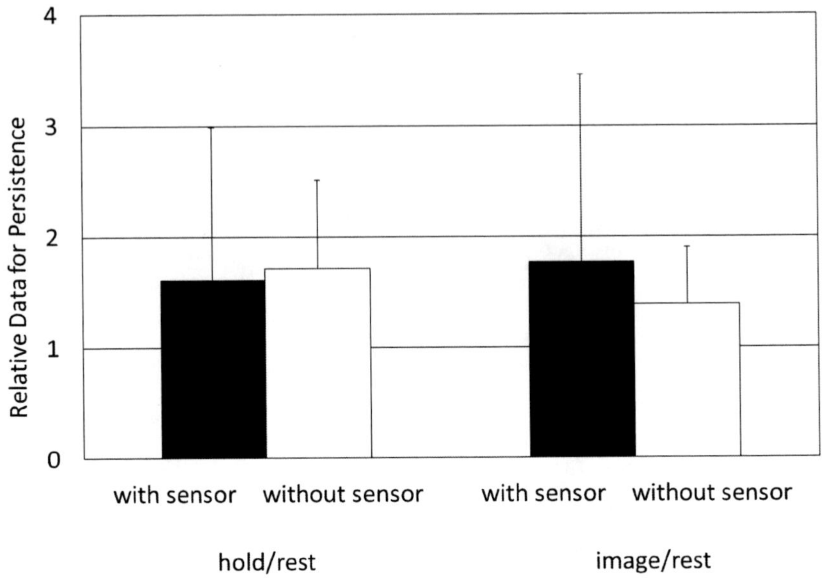

Figure 8. The relative persistence during the holding condition and during motor imagery under the "with sensor" and "without sensor" conditions.

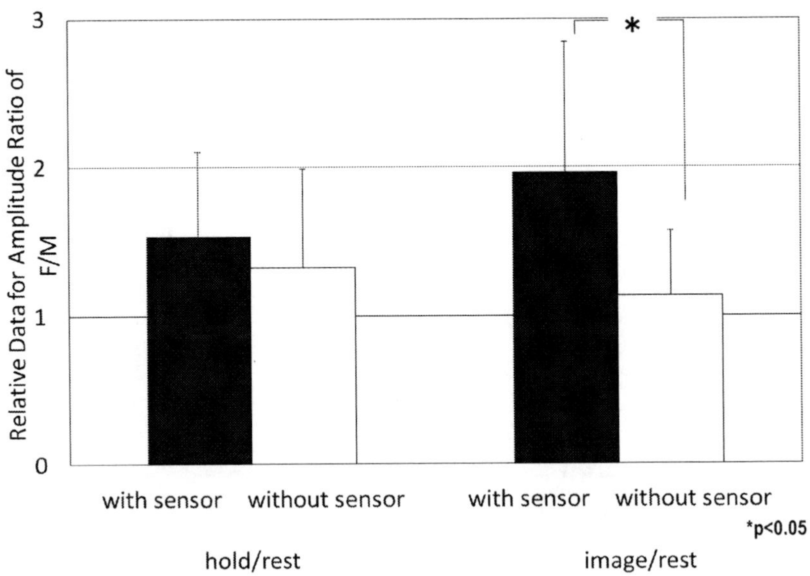

Figure 9. The relative F/M amplitude ratio during the holding condition and during motor imagery under "with sensor" and "without sensor" conditions.

2.4. Discussion

Research on motor imagery can be conducted using a variety of methods. With regard to MEPs obtained using TMS and single-photon emission computed tomography, it is presumed that motor imagery will increase excitability at the cerebral cortex level of the motor area, supplementary motor area, premotor region, and gyrus cinguli.

However, various studies reported the influence of motor imagery on the excitability of spinal neural function. Kasai et al. (1997) reported that the amplitude of the H-reflex of the radial flexor muscle during motor imagery with wrist flexion was not increased, whereas the amplitude of MEPs was increased. Oishi et al. (1994) reported that the amplitude of the H-reflex during motor imagery was decreased in a speed skater. These reports support the argument that motor imagery cannot increase the excitability of spinal neural function. Jeannerod (1995) reported that the amplitudes of the H-reflex and T-wave during pedaling with motor imagery were significantly greater than those during pedaling without motor imagery. Furthermore, because the increase in the amplitude of the T-wave during motor imagery was significantly greater than that of the H-reflex, the excitability of spinal neural function by motor imagery was affected by the excitability of α-motoneurons. Hale et al. (2003) reported that the amplitude of the H-reflex of the soleus muscle during motor imagery with ankle planter flexion under 40, 60, 80, and 100% MVC gradually increased with motor imagery training. These reports further support the theory that motor imagery is effective in exciting spinal neural function.

In the present study, to examine spinal neural function during motor imagery tasks, we analyzed the F-wave of the thenar muscles after stimulating the median nerve during motor imagery conditions with the sensor held between the thumb and index finger (motor imagery under the "with sensor" condition) and without the sensor held (motor imagery under the "without sensor" condition). The persistence and F/M amplitude ratio during motor imagery with or without the sensor were higher than those during relaxation. In particular, the persistence and amplitude ratio during motor imagery under the "with sensor" condition were significantly higher than those during motor imagery under the "without sensor" condition. Because the persistence and F/M amplitude ratio are indices of excitability of spinal neural function, motor imagery with or without the sensor facilitated spinal neural function.

The relative persistence and amplitude ratio during motor imagery under the "with sensor" condition were higher than those during motor imagery under the "without sensor" condition. We believe that the volume of the afferent pathways from proprioception and skin mechanoreceptors to the primary somatosensory cortex tends to increase more during motor imagery under the "with sensor" condition than during motor imagery under the "without sensor" condition.

Vargas et al. (2004) reported that a proprioceptive signal enhanced corticospinal excitability during motor imagery. However, Mizuguchi, Sakamoto, Muraoka, and Kanosue (2009) reported that the responsiveness of afferent mechanoreceptors to the primary somatosensory cortex did not change even during a combination of motor imagery of squeezing a ball and that of actually touching it. Therefore, the excitability of spinal neural function during motor imagery under the "with sensor" condition was caused by both proprioception and some modulation along the corticospinal pathway, including the primary motor cortex itself.

3. Excitability of Spinal Neural Function by Motor Imagery with Isometric Opponens Pollicis Activity: Influence of Vision during Motor Imagery (NeuroRehabilitation 34:725–729, 2014)

3.1. Purpose

In the present study, subjects were instructed to achieve 50% MVC by isometrically contracting the opponens pollicis muscle using a pinch meter to accurately track the number of movements on a monitor. The subjects were then asked to maintain the number of contractions on the display of the pinch meter by mental imaging. The patients were instructed to hold the sensor between their thumbs and index fingers and mimic the number of contractions displayed on the pinch meter while watching (eyes open) or not watching it (eyes closed). During these motor imagery conditions, we monitored the F-waves of the left thenar muscles after stimulating the left median nerve at the wrist. The F-wave data were obtained from the backfiring of the α-motoneurons after antidromic invasion of the propagated impulses across the axon hillock (Kimura, 1974). Its occurrence reflects excitability changes of the spinal motoneurons, as reported in patients with spasticity (Odusote & Eisen,

1979) and healthy subjects by isometric contraction (Suzuki, Fujiwara, & Takeda, 2013).

3.2. Material and Methods

3.2.1. Subjects

In total, 16 healthy volunteers (12 males and 4 females; mean age, 35.1 years) participated in this study. Written informed consent was obtained from all subjects. This study was approved by the Research Ethics Committee of Kansai University of Health Sciences (Osaka, Japan), and all experiments were conducted in accordance with the Declaration of Helsinki.

3.2.2. Methods

Subjects were comfortably positioned in a supine position while rotating both shoulders. The skin of the patients was prepared with an abrasive gel to maintain the impedance below 5 kΩ. A Viking Quest electromyography machine (Natus Medical Inc., CA, USA) was used to record the F-waves of the left thenar muscles with a pair of round disks attached (with collodion) to the skin over the abdomen of the thenar muscle and the metacarpophalangeal joint of the thumb after stimulating the left median nerve at the wrist at rest and under touch and motor imagery conditions. The stimulating electrodes comprised a cathode placed over the left median nerve 3 cm proximal to the palmar crease of the wrist and an anode placed 2 cm further proximally. The maximum stimulus was determined by delivering 0.2-ms square-wave pulses of increasing intensity to elicit the largest compound muscle action potentials. Supramaximal shocks, adjusted to a value of 20% higher than the maximal stimulus, were delivered at 0.5 Hz for F-wave acquisition. The bandwidth filter ranged from 2 Hz to 3 kHz.

In the resting condition, we tested the F-wave during relaxation and using motor imagery. First, we gauged MVC using a pinch meter by instructing the patients to isometrically contract their opponens pollicis muscles. The magnitude of MVC was numerically recorded on the display of the pinch meter. Next, the subjects were instructed to obtain 50% MVC by isometrically contracting their opponens pollicis muscles while maintaining the recorded value displayed on the pinch meter. Under motor imagery conditions, the subjects were asked to imagine maintaining the numerical value displayed on the pinch meter by holding the sensor between the thumb and index finger while either watching the display of the pinch meter (eyes open) or not watching it (eyes closed) (Figure 1).

The F-waves from 30 trials were analyzed with respect to persistence, the F/M amplitude ratio, and latency. Persistence was defined as the number of measurable F-wave responses divided by 30 trials of supramaximal stimulation. The F/M amplitude ratio was defined as the mean amplitude of all responses divided by the M-wave amplitude. Latency was defined as the mean time from stimulation to the onset of a measurable F-wave.

The Kruskal–Wallis, Mann–Whitney, and Bonferroni tests were used to compare results among the resting and motor imagery conditions under the conditions of eyes open or closed. A p-value of <0.05 was considered statistically significant.

For subjective comparisons after the test, we asked the patients whether imaging was easier with eyes open or closed. We compared the effects on the F-waves during motor imagery and by subjective evaluation.

3.3. Results

Persistence during motor imagery conditions with the eyes open and eyes closed parameters tended to increase compared with that observed at rest (Figure 10). Persistence remained unchanged under both conditions (Figure 10). The F/M amplitude ratio during motor imagery with the eyes open and eyes closed parameters was significantly greater than that observed at rest (Kruskal–Wallis test, Mann–Whitney test, and Bonferroni test; $*p < 0.05$) (Figure 11). There was no difference in the F/M amplitude ratio with the eyes open and eyes closed parameters (Figure 11). There was no significant difference in latency among the three conditions (Figure 12).

Almost all subjects (14/16) were adept at imaging using the eyes-open condition compared with the eyes-closed condition in subjective evaluations. However, there was no relationship between the F-wave data and subjective evaluations. In five of the 14 subjects, no changes were found in the F-waves using either the eyes-open or eyes-closed condition (Figure 13). A higher F-wave value was detected under the eyes-open condition in four subjects (Figure 14), and a higher F-wave value was detected in five subjects under the eyes-closed condition (Figure 15).

The remaining two subjects found it easier to foster an image without vision than with vision via subjective impression. However, the F/M amplitude ratio during imaging without vision was lower than that during imaging with vision.

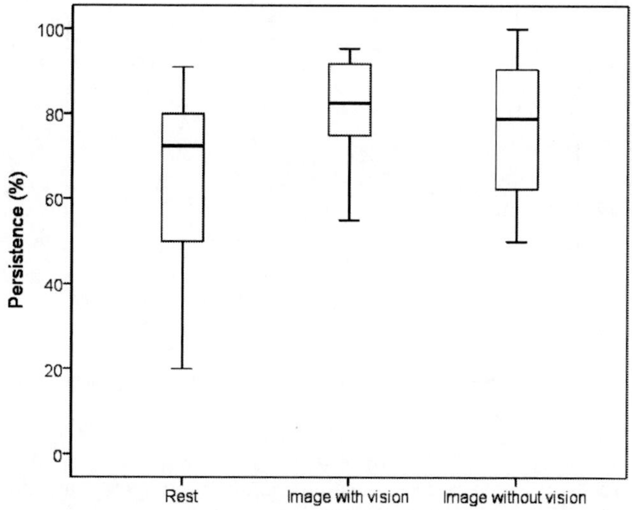

Figure 10. Persistence during resting and during imaging with and without vision.

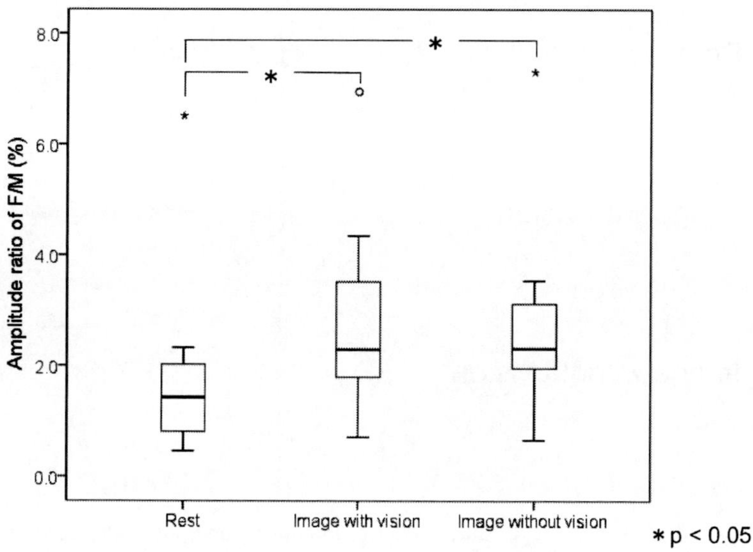

Figure 11. The F/M amplitude ratio during resting and during imaging with and without vision.

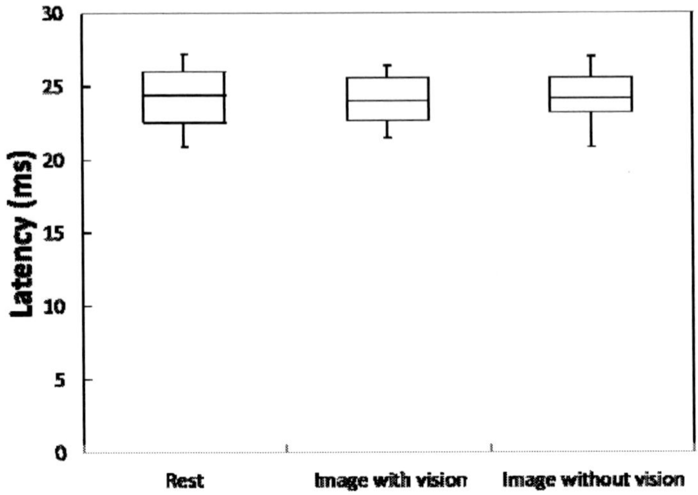

Figure 12. Latency of F-waves during resting and during imaging with and without vision.

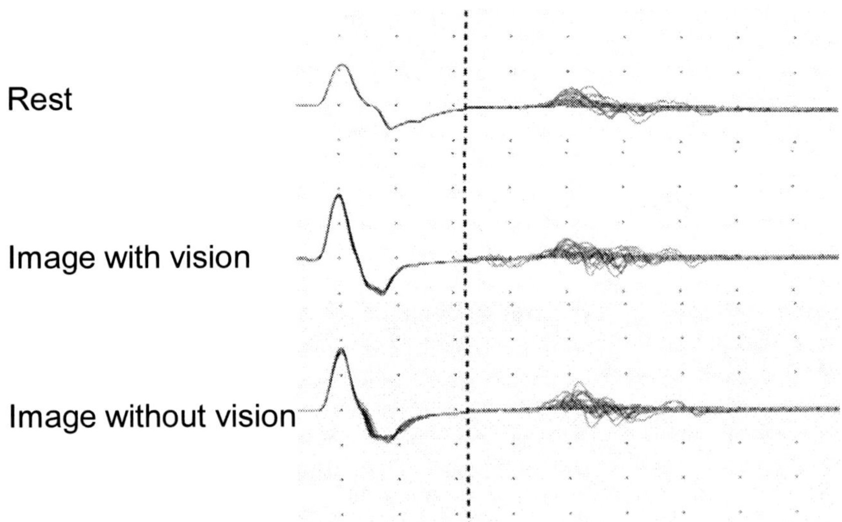

Figure 13. Typical F-waves during resting and during imaging with and without vision in 16 subjects (Cases with unchanged F-waves).

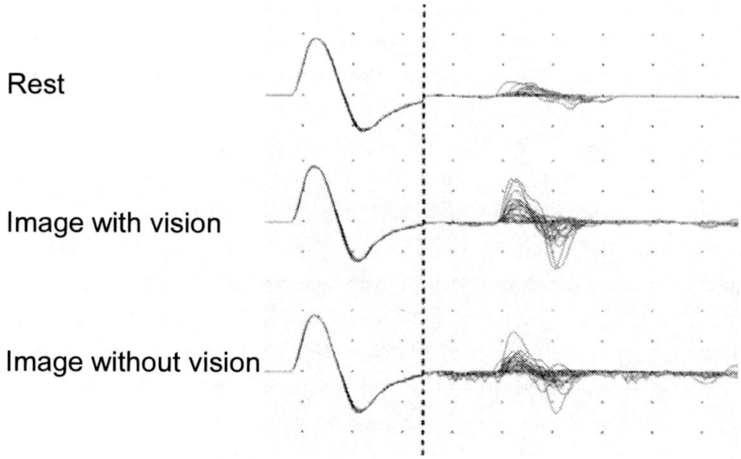

Figure 14. Typical F-waves during resting and during imaging with and without vision in 16 subjects (Cases with higher waves during visual imaging).

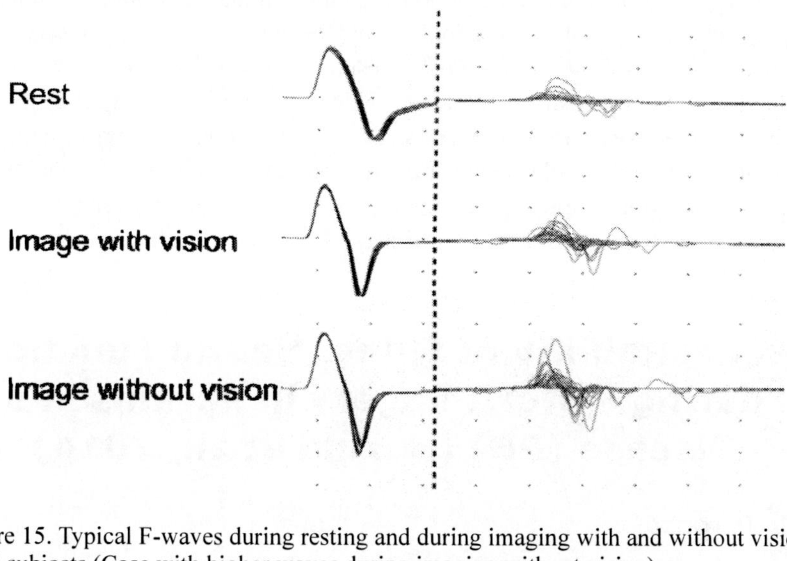

Figure 15. Typical F-waves during resting and during imaging with and without vision in 16 subjects (Case with higher waves during imaging without vision).

3.4. Discussion

In the present study, the subjects were asked whether imaging was easier with eyes open or closed. We hypothesized that imagery to maintain the number of concentrations recorded by the pinch meter with eyes open is more effective for the excitability of spinal neural function and that imagery used to maintain the number displayed on the pinch meter was easier for patients under the eyes-closed condition. The excitability of spinal neural function under both motor imagery conditions was increased compared with that in the resting condition, but there was no difference in the magnitudes of the excitability of spinal neural function under either condition.

For the motor imagery tasks in this study, the subjects were asked to imagine maintaining the number of contractions displayed on the pinch meter by holding the sensor between the thumb and index finger while watching the pinch meter display (eyes open) or not watching it (eyes closed). It is generally accepted that the observation of a movement influences the execution of that movement (Brass, Bekkering, Wohlschlaeger, & Prinz, 2000, Urgesi, Candidi, Fabbro, Romani, & Aglioti, 2006). When the pinch meter display was zero under the eyes-open condition, the subjects did not maintain the number displayed on the pinch meter. However, we hypothesized that during the excitability of spinal neural function by motor imagery while watching the display, the number of contractions would be higher than that observed via motor imagery without watching the display. On the basis of these results, merely watching the instrument using motor imagery was not significant.

The subjective evaluation results revealed that mental imaging with eyes open or closed had no significant influence on the excitability of spinal neural function. Therefore, motor imagery under these conditions for rehabilitation is not necessarily relevant for the excitability of spinal neural function.

4. Excitability of Spinal Neural Function during Motor Imagery in Parkinson's Disease (PD) (Suzuki et al., 2014)

4.1. Purpose

In this study, using the motor imagery conditions of our previous study, we tested the F-waves of the left thenar muscles after stimulating the left median nerve at the wrist in patients with PD.

4.2. Materials and Methods

4.2.1. Subjects

Ten patients with PD (2 males and 8 females; mean age, 63.9 ± 11.0 years; range, 38–81 years) participated in the study, and written informed consent was obtained from all subjects. This study was approved by the Research Ethics Committee of Kansai University of Health Sciences (Ref number 11-10). The experiments were conducted in accordance with the Declaration of Helsinki.

4.2.2. F-Waves during Motor Imagery (Figure 1)

Subjects were positioned comfortably in a supine position with external rotation of both shoulder joints. The skin was prepared with abrasive gel to maintain the impedance below 5 KΩ. A Viking Quest electromyography machine (Natus Medical Inc., CA, USA) was used to record the F-waves. We tested the F-waves of the left thenar muscles using a pair of disks attached (with collodion) to the skin over the belly and the bones of the metacarpophalangeal joint of the thumb after stimulating the left median nerve at the wrist at rest and under touch and motor imagery conditions. The stimulating electrodes comprised a cathode placed over the left median nerve 3 cm proximal to the palmar crease of the wrist joint and an anode placed 2 cm further proximally. The maximal stimulus was determined by delivering 0.2-ms square-wave pulses of increasing intensity to elicit the largest compound muscle action potentials. Supramaximal shocks (adjusted up to the value of 20% higher than the maximal stimulus) were delivered at 0.5 Hz for the acquisition of F-waves. The bandwidth filter ranged from 2 Hz to 3 kHz.

In the resting condition, we tested the F-wave that elicited no EMG signal from the left thenar muscles during relaxation. In the holding condition, the subject held the sensor of the pinch meter between the thumb and index finger. For the motor imagery condition, subjects first learned 50% MVC by isometrically contracting the opponens pollicis muscle while holding the sensor of the pinch meter. Specifically, the magnitude of MVC was numerically recorded on the display of the pinch meter. Next, the subjects were instructed to obtain 50% MVC by isometrically contracting their opponens pollicis muscles while maintaining the display value recorded on the pinch meter for 1 min. Finally, the subjects were asked to imagine the contraction while holding the pinch meter and sensor between the thumb and index finger (motor imagery under the "with sensor" condition) and, on a different day, while not holding the sensor (motor imagery under the "without sensor" condition).

4.2.3. Data Analysis

The F-waves from 30 trials were analyzed with respect to persistence, the F/M amplitude ratio, and latency. Persistence was defined as the number of measurable F-wave responses divided by 30 trials of supramaximal stimulation. The F/M amplitude ratio was defined as the mean amplitude of all responses divided by the amplitude of the M-wave. Latency was defined as the mean latency from the time of stimulation to the onset of a measurable F-wave. The statistical analysis for normal distribution was performed using the Komogorov–Smirnov and Shapiro–Wilk tests. From these results, because the data were not recognized as showing normal distribution, the Wilcoxon test was used to compare results between resting and the other conditions.

4.3. Results

Persistence during motor imagery under the "with sensor" condition was significantly better compared with that at rest (n = 10, z = 2.2509, p = 0.0244, Wilcoxon's test, Figure 16).

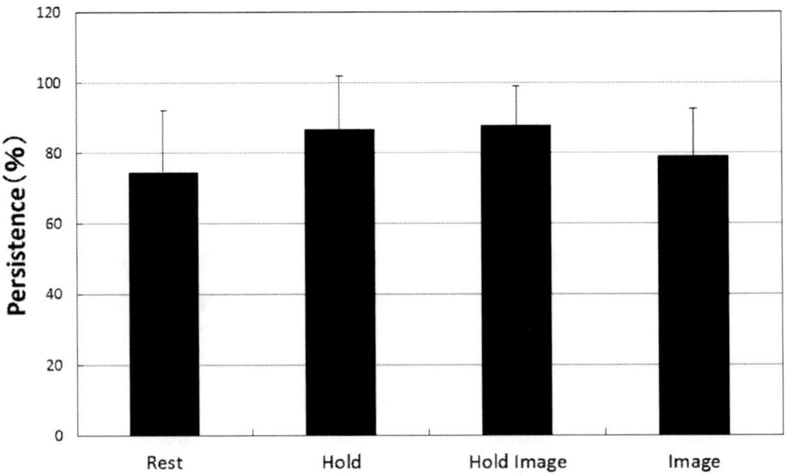

Figure 16. Persistence during resting, holding, and motor imagery under the "with sensor" condition and motor imagery under the "without sensor" condition. Hold Image: motor imagery under the "with sensor" condition. Image: motor imagery under the "without sensor" condition.

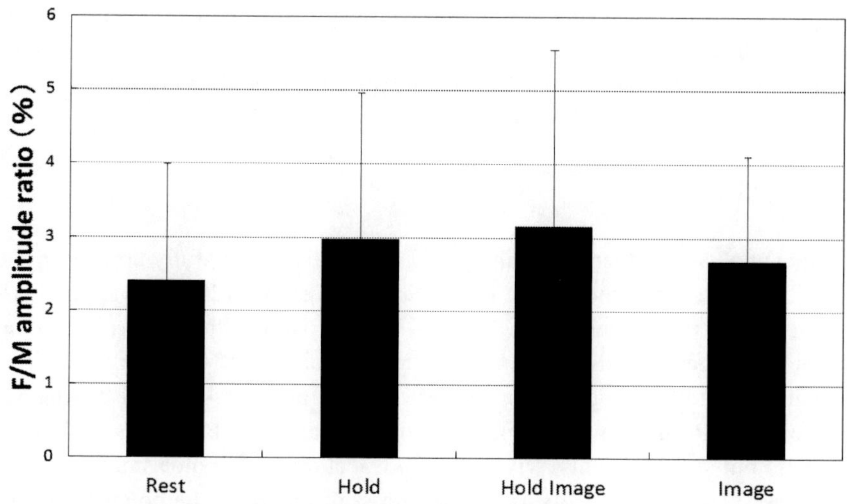

Figure 17. The F/M amplitude ratios during resting, holding, and motor imagery under the "with sensor" condition and motor imagery under the "without sensor" condition. Hold Image: motor imagery in the "with sensor" condition. Image: motor imagery in the "without sensor" condition.

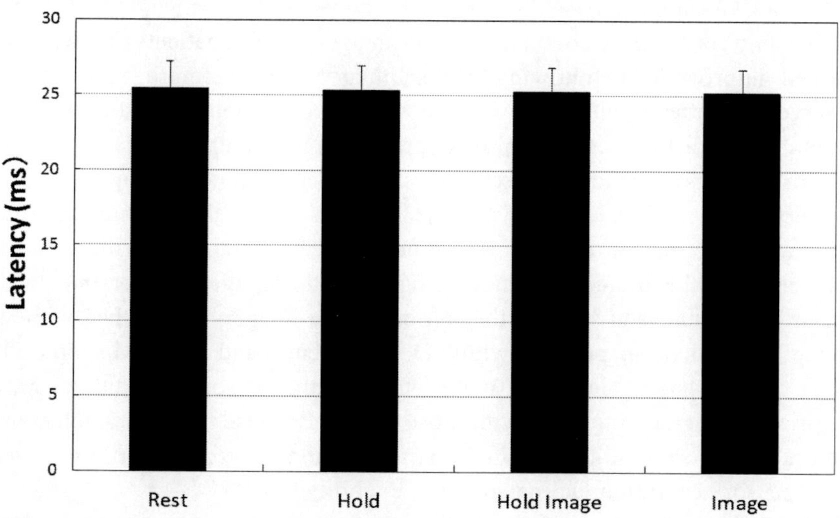

Figure 18. Latency during resting, holding, and motor imagery under the "with sensor" condition and motor imagery under the "without sensor" condition. Hold Image: motor imagery under the "with sensor" condition. Image: motor imagery under the "without sensor" condition.

There were no significant differences in persistence among all other conditions (Figure 16). The F/M amplitude ratio during motor imagery under the "with sensor" condition was significantly greater compared with that at rest ($n = 10$, $z = 2.1915$, $p = 0.0284$, Wilcoxon's test, Figure 17). There were no significant differences in latency among all three conditions (Figure 18).

4.4. Discussion

It is unclear whether motor imagery can also be successfully applied in the rehabilitation of patients with PD. Heremans et al. (2011) evaluated 14 patients with PD (Hoehn and Yahr 1-3) and 14 healthy controls via an extensive imagery ability assessment battery consisting of two questionnaires, the Chaotic Motor Imagery Assessment battery and a test based on mental chronometry. Patients with PD performed the imagery tasks more slowly than controls, but most patients' vividness and accuracy of motor imagery were well preserved. These results are promising with regard to the potential use of motor imagery practice in the rehabilitation of patients with PD. However, Yaguez et al. (1999) reported on 12 patients with PD who received 10 min of motor imagery training followed by a motor practice phase. In addition, a test battery for visual imagery abilities was administered to investigate the possible relationship between visual and motor imagery. The patients showed no marked improvement following motor imagery. Furthermore, the deficits observed in patients with PD may also be related to their limited attentional resources and difficulties in employing predictive motor strategies.

In the present study, to examine spinal neural function during motor imagery tasks for PD, we analyzed the F-waves of the thenar muscles after stimulating the median nerve during motor imagery conditions with a sensor held between the thumb and index finger (motor imagery under the "with sensor" condition) and without the sensor (motor imagery under the "without sensor" condition) in patients with PD. Persistence and the F/M amplitude ratio during motor imagery under the "with sensor" condition were significantly higher compared with those at rest. Because these parameters are indices of the excitability of spinal neural function, motor imagery under the "with sensor" condition facilitated this excitability.

We believe that the volume of afferent pathways from proprioception and skin mechanoreceptors to the primary somatosensory cortex tends to increase more during the touch and motor imagery conditions under the "with sensor" condition than under other conditions.

Vargas et al. (2004) reported that a proprioceptive signal enhanced corticospinal excitability during motor imagery. However, Mizuguchi, et al.

(2009) reported that the responsiveness of the afferent mechanoreceptors to the primary somatosensory cortex did not change even during the combination of the motor imagery of squeezing a ball and that of actually touching it. Because only the touch condition tended to increase spinal neural function in the above study, the excitability of spinal neural function during motor imagery under the "with sensor" condition was caused by both proprioception and a degree of modulation along the corticospinal pathway, including the primary motor cortex itself.

From this study, we believe that the motor imagery task under the "with sensor" condition involving isometric opponens pollicis activity was effective because of the excitability of spinal neural function in patients with PD, as previously observed in healthy subjects (Suzuki et al., 2013). Suzuki et al. (2013) reported that motor imagery under the "with sensor" and "without sensor" conditions at approximately 50% MVC of the opponens pollicis without overt motor output increased the excitability of spinal neural output to the thenar muscles in healthy subjects. In healthy subjects, motor imagery at approximately 50% MVC of the opponens pollicis was effective. However, both Suzuki et al. (2013) and the present study revealed that in order to use motor imagery task in the rehabilitation of patients with PD, movement preparation for a motor imagery task is extremely important.

The present study had several limitations. We used motor imagery tasks involving isometric opponens pollicis activity in patients with PD. In addition, we did not utilize other motor imagery tasks in such patients. In the future, we would like to investigate several motor imagery tasks in patients with PD.

Conclusion

Motor imagery under the "with sensor" and "without sensor" conditions at approximately 50% MVC of the opponens pollicis without overt motor output increased the excitability of spinal neural output to the thenar muscles. Because the relative data for the persistence and F/M amplitude ratio during motor imagery under the "with sensor" condition were higher than those during that under the "without sensor" condition, the movement preparation for a motor imagery task involving 50% MVC of the opponens pollicis is extremely important.

Motor imagery while maintaining 50% MVC of the opponens pollicis muscle without overt motor output with a subject's eyes open or closed increased the excitability of spinal neural output to the subject's thenar muscles. There was no significant difference in the excitability of spinal neural function by motor imagery under these conditions. The subjective evaluations illustrated that motor imagery with the subject's eyes open or closed had no effect on motor imagery.

Motor imagery under both the "with sensor" and "without sensor" conditions at approximately 50% MVC of the opponens pollicis without overt motor output increased the excitability of spinal neural output to the thenar muscles in 10 patients with PD (2 males and 8 females; mean age, 64 years). Because persistence and the F/M amplitude ratio during motor imagery under the "with sensor" condition were significantly higher compared with those at rest, movement preparation for a motor imagery task involving 50% MVC of the opponens pollicis is extremely important.

Declaration of Competing Interests: The authors declare that there are no conflicts of interest.

References

Brass, M., Bekkering, H., Wohlschlaeger, A. & Prinz, W. (2000). Compatibility between observed and executed finger movements: comparing symbolic, spatial and imitative cues. *Brain and Cognition*, 44, 124-143.

Hale, B. S., Raglin, J. S. & Koceja, D. M. (2003). Effect of mental imagery of a motor task on the Hoffmann reflex. *Behavioural Brain Research,* 142, 1-87.

Hashimoto, R. & Rothwell, J. C. (1999). Dynamic changes in corticospinal excitability during motor imagery. *Experimental Brain Research,* 125, 75-81.

Heremans, E., Feys, P., Nieuwboer, A., et al. (2011). Motor imagery ability in patients with early- and mid-stage Parkinson disease. *Neurorehabilitation and Neural Repair,* 25, 168-177

Jeannerod, M. (1995). Mental imagery in the motor context. *Neuropsychologia,* 33, 1419-1432.

Kasai, T., Kawai, S., Kawanishi, M. & Yahagi, S. (1997). Evidence for facilitation of motor evoked potentials (MEPs) induced by motor imagery. *Brain Research,* 744, 147-150.

Kimura, J. (1974). F-wave velocity in the central segment of the median and ulnar nerves. A study in normal subjects and in patients with Charcot-Marie-Tooth disease. *Neurology,* 24, 539-546.

Li, S., Latash, M. L. & Zatsiorsky, V. M. (2004). Effects of motor imagery on finger force responses to transcranial magnetic stimulation. Brain Research. *Cognitive Brain Research,* 20, 273-280.

Mizuguchi, N., Sakamoto, M., Muraoka, T. & Kanosue, K. (2009). Influence of touching an object on corticospinal excitability during motor imagery. *Experimental Brain Research,* 196, 529-535.

Odusote, K. & Eisen, A. (1979). An electrophysiological quantitation of the cubital tunnel syndrome. *The Canadian Journal of Neurological Sciences,* 6, 403-410.

Oishi, K., Kimura, M., Yasukawa, T., Yoneda, T. & Maeshima, T. (1994). Amplitude reduction of H-reflex during mental movement simulation in elite athletes. *Behavioural Brain Research,* 62, 55-61.

Pascual-Leone, A., Nguyet, D., Cohen, L. G., Brasil-Neto, J. P., Cammarota, A. & Hallet M. (1995). Modulation of muscle responses evoked by transcranial magnetic stimulation during the acquisition of new fine motor skills. *Journal of Neurophysiology,* 74, 1037-1045.

Ryding, E., Decety, J., Sjoholm, H., Stenberg, G. & Ingvar, D. H. (1993). Motor imagery activates the cerebellum regionally. A SPECT rCBF study with 99mTc-HMPAO. Brain Research. *Cognitive Brain Research,* 1, 94-99.

Stevens, J. A. & Stoykov, M. E. (2003). Using motor imagery in the rehabilitation of hemiparesis. *Archives of Physical Medicine and Rehabilitation,* 84, 1090-1092.

Suzuki, T., Bunnno, Y., Onigata, C., Tani, M. & Uragami, S. (2013) Excitability of spinal neural function during several motor imagery tasks involving isometric opponens pollicis activity. *NeuroRehabilitation,* 33, 171-176.

Suzuki, T., Bunnno, Y., Onigata, C., Tani, M. & Uragami, S. (2014). Excitability of spinal neural function by motor imagery with isometric opponens pollicis activity: influence of vision during motor imagery. *NeuroRehabilitation,* 34, 725-729.

Suzuki, T., Bunnno, Y., Onigata, C., Tani, M., Uragami, S. & Yoshida S. (2014). Excitability of spinal neural function during motor imagery in Parkinson's disease. *Functional Neurology,* 22, 1-5.

Suzuki, T., Bunno, Y., Onigata, C., et al. (2013). Excitability of spinal neural function during several motor imagery tasks involving isometric opponens pollicis activity. *NeuroRehabilitation,* 33, 171-176.

Suzuki, T., Fujiwara, T. & Takeda, I. (1993). Excitability of the spinal motor neuron pool and F-wave during isometric ipsilateral and contralateral contraction. *Physiotherapy Theory and Practice,* 9, 19-24.

Urgesi, C., Candidi, M., Fabbro, F., Romani, M., Aglioti, S. M. (2006). Motor facilitation during action observation: topographic mapping of the target muscle and influence of the onlooker's posture, *The European Journal of Neuroscience,* 23, 2522-2530.

Vargas, C. D., Olivier, E., Craighero, L., Fadiga, L., Duhamel, J. R. & Sirigu, A. (2004). The influence of hand posture on corticospinal excitability during motor imagery: a transcranial magnetic stimulation study. *Cerebral Cortex,* 14, 1200-1206.

Yaguez, L., Canavan, A. G., Lange, H. W., et al. (1999). Motor learning by imagery is differentially affected in Parkinson's and Huntington's diseases. *Behavioural Brain Research,* 102, 115-127.

In: Motor Imagery
Editor: Brandon M. Garcia

ISBN: 978-1-63483-125-3

Chapter 2

Motor Imagery in Children with Developmental Coordination Disorder

Priscila Caçola*[*], *PhD
Director, Developmental Motor Cognition Lab, Assistant Professor, Department of Kinesiology, University of Texas at Arlington, Arlington, TX, US

Abstract

Developmental Coordination Disorder (DCD) is a disorder that defines children with problems in their motor coordination development despite their intelligence levels and impacts about 2-7% of school-age children. While the degree of motor impairment varies, common symptoms of the disorder include marked delays in achieving motor milestones and clumsiness, normally associated with poor balance, coordination, and handwriting skills. These difficulties associated with motor learning and control may last well into adolescence and adulthood. In this chapter, I will provide a description of how children with DCD are said to have difficulties with motor imagery (MI), i.e., the ability to mentally representing motor behavior, planning and generating an

[*] EMAIL: cacola@uta.edu.

accurate visuospatial representation of an intended action, and coupling sensory information with appropriate motor actions. The neurocognitive perspective states that this problem results from an underlying deficit in generating and/or monitoring internal models of action, termed the internal modeling deficit (IMD) hypothesis. This hypothesis has been largely accepted as one of the likely causes of the motor skill difficulties presented in DCD. The understanding of the IMD hypothesis and how children with DCD use motor imagery offers practical applications for the understanding of screening, diagnostic, and rehabilitation protocols in physical therapy. Here, I will also explore such clinical implications and provide suggestions and strategies for rehabilitation in these children.

Keywords: Developmental Coordination Disorder (DCD), children, motor imagery (MI), rehabilitation

Introduction

Motor imagery (MI) is defined as an internal rehearsal or reenactment of movements from a first-person perspective without any overt physical movement. It is well known that motor imagery has the potential to promote greater insight to the development of action planning, and because of that, it is now considered a fundamental topic of study in the field of motor behavior (Gabbard, Caçola, & Lee, 2013). Motor imagery has also been linked to deficits observed in individuals with Developmental Coordination Disorder (DCD). Developmental Coordination Disorder (DCD) is a disorder that defines children with problems in their motor coordination development despite their intelligence levels, impacting about 2-7% of school-age children (American Psychiatric Association, 2013). Common symptoms include marked delays in achieving motor milestones and clumsiness, typically associated with poor balance, coordination, and especially handwriting skills. More importantly, DCD is considered to be one of the major health problems among school-aged children worldwide (Cairney, Hay, Faught, & Hawes, 2005, Green, Baird, & Sugden, 2006, Henderson & Henderson, 2002; Polatajko & Cantin, 2005).

Here, I will explore Developmental Coordination Disorder as a condition, and describe the studies that link MI to the causes of motor skill difficulties presented in DCD. The understanding of motor imagery in this special population will provide practical applications for the conception, understanding, and refinement of screening, diagnostic, and rehabilitation protocols in physical therapy. I will also explore such clinical implications and provide suggestions and strategies for rehabilitation in this condition.

Developmental Coordination Disorder (DCD)

As previously mentioned, DCD is defined as a neurodevelopmental condition characterized by poor motor proficiency that interferes with an individual's activities of daily living (Rivilis et al., 2011). This disorder defines children who, for no medical reasons, fail to acquire adequate motor skills despite their intelligence levels (Zoia, Barnett, Wilson, & Hill, 2006). The movements of children with DCD are often described as "clumsy" and "uncoordinated," and frequently lead to performance difficulties that typically developing children perform easily. Campbell, Missiuna, and Vaillancourt (2012) state that children with DCD are not just low in athletic ability; they struggle to perform the everyday activities that most of us take for granted - zipping a knapsack, tying shoes, using scissors, or buttering bread. Other general difficulties commonly associated with DCD include poor fine and gross motor control, speech fluency, abnormal muscle tone (hypo/ hypertonia), poor body awareness, and gross motor sequencing. According to Caçola (2014), those general complications can be observed when children with DCD attempt to plan a motor task, organize movements, perform a coordinated action, and adjust movements when demands change, such as moving fast to catch a ball.

Gibbs, Appleton, and Appleton (2007) described DCD as a ''hidden problem,'' with an estimated prevalence as high as 10% in school-aged children. In general, estimates of 2% to 7% are more likely (American Psychiatric Association, 2013), implying that most school classes have at least one affected child. Estimates suggest it affects four times more males than females, and according to Holsti, Grunau, and Whitfield (2002), children born prematurely and/or with extremely low birth weights are at a significantly increased risk of demonstrating DCD. Interestingly, difficulties associated with motor learning and control can last well into adolescence and adulthood (see reviews by Bo & Lee, 2013 and Zwicker, Missiuna, Harris, & Boyd, 2012).

Approximately 25% of children with DCD are referred and diagnosed before starting school. The remaining 75% are referred during the first few years in primary school. Presentation at this age includes persistence of the problems noted in the preschool years, such as slow, immature and laborious handwriting and difficulties in copying from the blackboard. According to Missiuna, Rivard, and Pollock (2004), handwriting problems are readily apparent to classroom teachers, but might be only the tip of the iceberg for children who have significant DCD, indicating that other motor coordination difficulties are present. This marked impairment in the development of motor coordination is the first item on the assessment criteria created by the Diagnostic and Statistical Manual of Mental Disorders, Fifth Edition (DSM-5). In this document, DCD is characterized as a Neurodevelopmental Disorder, and has three items that must be followed for a correct diagnosis: A. Motor performance that is substantially below expected levels, given the person's chronologic age and previous opportunities for skill acquisition. The poor motor performance may manifest as coordination problems, poor balance, clumsiness, dropping or bumping into things; marked delays in achieving developmental motor milestones (e.g., walking, crawling, sitting) or in the acquisition of basic motor skills (e.g., catching, throwing, kicking, running, jumping, hopping, cutting, coloring, printing, writing); B. The disturbance in Criterion A, without accommodations, significantly interferes with activities of daily living or academic achievement; and C. The disturbance is not due to a general medical condition (e.g., cerebral palsy, hemiplegia, or muscular dystrophy). In addition, the diagnostician determines that the onset of the symptoms is in the early developmental period. In essence, a diagnosis is not only focused on motor coordination difficulties, but also on ruling out all other conditions that might be the cause of movement difficulties.

It is important for physical therapists to be aware that movements in children with DCD have three main characteristics (Caçola, 2014): (1) They are slower. Overall, in comparison with typically developing children, children will perform movements at a slower pace. If facing time constraints, DCD children will be even slower (the anxiety and pressure can take over, slowing down the movement even more) then when they are not in timed situations. Giving them more time (or not focus on the time it takes to perform a movement task at all, e.g., handwriting) can help; (2) Movements are less accurate. In general, movements of children with DCD are more variable, which makes difficult for children to perform tasks that require a high degree of precision; and (3) Movements typically take more "effort." Children with DCD use a greater rate of their capacity in order to perform than typically developing children. These three characteristics are always present in movements performed in children with DCD, and it is crucial to remember those three features (slower, less accurate, more effort) in order to understand and help children accomplish tasks.

Internal Modeling Deficit Hypothesis (IMD)

More specific to the present chapter, children with DCD are said to have difficulties with motor imagery (MI), i.e., the ability to mentally representing motor behavior (see review by Gabbard & Bobbio, 2011), planning and generating an accurate visuospatial representation of an intended action (Maruff et al., 1999), and coupling sensory information with appropriate motor actions (Mackenzie et al., 2008).

The neurocognitive perspective states that this problem results from an underlying deficit in generating and/or monitoring internal models of action, termed the internal modeling deficit (IMD) hypothesis (e.g., Deconinick, Spitaels, Fias, & Lenoir, 2009; Lewis, Vance, Maruff, Wilson, & Cairney, 2008; Pettit et al., 2008; Van Waelvelde et al., 2006; Williams, Thomas, Maruff, Butson, & Wilson, 2006; Williams, Thomas, Maruff, & Wilson, 2008; Williams, Omizzolo, Galea, & Vance, 2013, Wilson et al., 2004). Internal models provide stability to the motor system by predicting the outcome of movements before slow, sensori-motor feedback becomes available (Wolpert, 1997), providing a means of rapid online correction (Hyde and Wilson, 2011a,b). According to this premise, children with DCD have significant limitations in their ability to accurately generate and utilize internal models of motor planning and control (i.e., motor imagery). Dysfunction to this mode of control would severely impact the motor learning capabilities of a child, consistent with the profile of performance we see in children with DCD. These children are characterized by slow, effortful, and inaccurate movements, and are regarded as being overly dependent on visual feedback (Wilson et al., 2013).

Several experiments using MI paradigms have found differences between performance of TD children and children with DCD, reinforcing the IMD hypothesis. For example, TD children tend to be affected by biomechanical and time constraints of actual movements when performing MI tasks, while children with DCD are not as affected. While their actual movements are influenced by speed-accuracy trade-offs, their imagined movements are not (Wilson et al., 2001). Other paradigms including covert orienting of visuospatial attention (e.g., Tsai et al., 2009; Wilmut et al., 2007; Wilson and Maruff, 1999; Wilson et al., 1997), imagined or simulated pointing (e.g., Lewis et al., 2008; Maruff et al., 1999), mental rotation of limb-versus object-based stimuli (e.g., Williams et al., 2006, 2008, 2012), predictive control of eye movements (e.g., Katschmarsky et al., 2001; Langaas et al., 1998), grip force and anticipatory postural adjustments (e.g., Jover et al., 2010; Jucaite et al., 2003; Pereira et al., 2001), and studies on the rapid online control of reaching movements (e.g., Hyde and Wilson, 2011a,b) have also supported the IMD hypothesis.

A recent systematic literature review (Adams, Lust, Wilson, & Steenbergen, 2015) has examined the available evidence for the IMD hypothesis. The authors identified 48 relevant articles and categorized them according to the effector system involved in the evaluation of motor control, indicating that individuals with DCD have demonstrated compromised control of 1) overt and covert eye movements, 2) dynamic postural control, 3) manual control for tasks that vary in complexity, and 4) motor imagery of manual and whole-body postures. In this chapter, we are only focusing on the "motor imagery" aspect of the IMD hypothesis, and showing that there is enough evidence within this aspect to significantly support the IMD hypothesis as a cause of DCD.

Motor Imagery (MI)

MI is described as an active cognitive process during which the representation of a specific action is internally reproduced in working memory without any overt motor output from a first-person perspective (Decety & Grèzes, 1999). From another perspective, MI is defined as an internal rehearsal or reenactment of movements from a first-person perspective without any overt physical movement. MI is also considered a form of motor cognition; i.e., the cognitive level of action processing. Motor cognition takes into account recognizing, anticipating, predicting and production of actions. Steenbergen, Van Nimwegen, and Crajé (2007) have suggested that MI may be a necessary prerequisite for motor planning. In addition, MI provides a window into the process of action representation; that is, it reflects an internal action representation (Jeannerod, 2001; Munzert et al., 2009). In other words, MI tasks can provide an applied perspective to the study of action representation.

Typically, MI is studied from three different perspectives: Accuracy, timing, and vividness of the imagery. The first dimension relates to precision of the imagery, and is explored by tasks for which subjects imagine a movement in order to make a decision about some visual stimuli (e.g., mental rotation tasks of hand/numbers; reach to grasp tasks). The second dimension involves timing of imagined actions. It is assumed that motor execution and MI involve similar central processes (Jeannerod, 2001). Therefore the duration of execution and imagination should be nearly the same, as noted by the mental chronometry paradigm. The third dimension refers to the vividness of motor representation, the clarity of the image or the sensations perceived during MI. Questionnaires like the Kinesthetic and Visual Imagery Questionnaire (KVIQ; Malouin et al., 2007) or the Vividness of Movement Imagery Questionnaire (VMIQ, Isaac, Marks & Russel, 1986) are used to measure MI vividness.

Many studies have examined the development of MI within children (see Gabbard, 2009 for a review). It has been shown that children as young as 5 years of age are able to mentally rotate hands (e.g., Funk, Brugger, & Wilkening; 2005; Molina, Tijus, & Jouen, 2008).This ability is gradually refining through development, with 11-year-old children showing significantly higher accuracy than 7- and 8-year-olds (Butson, Hyde, Steenbergen, & Williams; 2014; Toussaint, Tahej, Thibaut, Possamai, & Badets, 2013) in a motor imagery accuracy task. Other studies have indicated clear age differences with significant improvements occurring at seven and eight years of age (Caeyenberghs et al., 2009), which is possibly related to the notion that with 7-year-olds, motor imagery emerges from their own sensorimotor sensation (Molina et al., 2008). In fact, it is well-known that motor imagery capacity depends directly on real motor activity of the children (Caeyenberghs, et al., 2009), which sets the stage for the IMD hypothesis as a possible cause or mechanism of Developmental Coordination Disorder.

Motor Imagery Studies in DCD

Wilson and colleagues have shown across a series of studies that children with DCD display atypical reaction times (Noten et al., 2014 and Wilson et al., 2004) and increased errors (Williams et al., 2006 and Williams et al., 2011) relative to age-matched controls when performing limb and body rotation tasks. Interestingly, Williams et al. (2006) showed that while MI appears to be compromised in DCD, non-motoric forms of imagery (e.g., visual imagery) remain preserved. Williams et al. (2008) later showed that MI deficits in DCD become more pronounced as the severity of the disorder increases. Indeed, in severe cases of DCD, performance deficits on the hand rotation task appear to mirror those found in children with severe neurological deficits of movement including congenital spastic hemiplegia (Williams et al., 2011).

Maruff, Wilson, Trebilcock and Currie (1999) examined the chronometry of real and imagined movements using a visually-guided pointing task with a Fitts' law paradigm [speed for accuracy trade-offs that occur as target size varied for both real and imagined performance]. Performance of the control group conformed to Fitts' law. In the DCD group, only real movements conformed. The researchers concluded that children with DCD shows an impaired ability to generate internal representations of volitional movements – this impairment was defined as an internal modelling deficit (IMD) hypothesis.

Wilson and colleagues (2004) further tested this hypothesis using a mental rotation paradigm. Participants included children with DCD and controls; both 10 years of age. The task required children to judge the handedness (side) of single-hand images that were presented at angles between 0° and 180° at 45° intervals in either direction. Responses of the control children conformed to the typical pattern of mental rotation: a moderate trade-off between response time and angle of rotation. However, the response pattern for the DCD group was less typical; that is, there was a small trade-off function. Response accuracy did not differ between groups. Researchers suggested that children with DCD, unlike controls, do not automatically engage MI when performing mental rotation, but rely on an alternative object-based strategy. It was concluded that these children manifest a reduced ability to make imagined transformations from an egocentric or first-person perspective.

Van Waelvelde and collegues (2006) also reported evidence indicating the children with DCD have problems with internal representation of action. The researchers used a rhythmic finger-tapping task in combination with a jumping and a drawing activity to evaluate children with DCD and a matched control group. In children with DCD, an increased temporal variability was found with finger tapping when compared with the controls. Errors in time correlated significantly with the jumping and drawing task, while errors in space did not. It was concluded that children with DCD have more problems in building up an internal representation of the movement. The researchers went on to suggest that deficits in temporal movement parameterization might be one of the underlying causes of poor motor performance in some children with DCD.

In 2006, Williams, Thomas, Maruff, Butson and Wilson used a mental rotation paradigm with typically developing and children with DCD (ages 7 to 11) to continue exploring this hypothesis. Groups were asked to complete hand rotation tasks with and without explicit imagery instructions. In the instruction condition, participants were asked to imagine their own hand in the position of the stimulus. Overall, there were no significant differences between the DCD and control groups when the hand task was completed without explicit instructions, on either response time or accuracy. However, when imagery instructions were introduced, the controls were significantly more accurate than the DCD group, indicating that children with DCD were unable to benefit from explicit cuing. In addition to the hand tasks, participants also completed an alphanumeric task, and as predicted, no group difference was found. In summary, results indicated partial support for the IMD hypothesis with DCD children.

In a subsequent study (2008), Williams et al. examined MI ability in DCD children aged 7- to 11 years with the intent to determine whether children with varying degrees of motor impairment differed in their ability to perform MI tasks. DCD children were split into two groups (DCD severe [DCD-S] and DCD mild [DCD-M]) and compared to age matched controls. Participants performed two MI tasks – hand (performed without and with specific imagery instructions) and whole-body rotation. Results indicated that children in the DCD-S group had a generalized MI deficit, in that they were less accurate across tasks than controls (and the DCD-M group on the hand task) and showed little benefit when given specific imagery instructions. The DCD-M group appeared capable of performing simpler MI transformations, but was less successful as task complexity increased. Unlike the DCD-S group, the DCD-M group did show some benefit from specific imagery instructions with increases in accuracy on the hand task. The findings suggested that a MI deficit does exist in many children with DCD but that its degree can vary. That is, factors such as individual ability level and task complexity appear to be linked to the deficit.

Also in 2008, Lewis et al. examined movement durations for real and imagined movements in a visually guided pointing task in children aged 8- to 12 years old and (similar to previous studies noted) found that the DCD group demonstrated an inability to generate imagined movements that was not present in the typically developing participants. That same year, Deconinck, Spitaels, Fias, and Lenior (2008) investigated the IMD hypothesis with 9-year-old children with DCD using a mental (hand / letters) rotation paradigm using various stimulus orientations. Results indicated that children with DCD were generally slower and made more errors than the typically developing control sample. As expected, both groups displayed fewer errors and faster responses in the letter, compared to hand conditions. This complements the reasoning that the motor task requires additional resources compared to the visual (letter) task. The researchers concluded that both groups did use an imagery strategy; however, judgments of the DCD group seem to be compromised by a less well-defined internal model. From another perspective, motor imagery has shown to be affected in children with DCD only in conditions with complex task constraints (i.e., rotation of hand stimuli presented in palm view in a mental rotation task of hands) (Noten et al., 2014).

More recently, Williams, Omizzolo, Galea, and Vance (2013) investigated whether the MI deficits found in children with DCD were linked to inattention, seen in about 50% of these children. The performance of four groups of children aged 7-12 years was compared using an imagined pointing task and a hand rotation task. Groups consisted of children with ADHD, ADHD + DCD, DCD alone, and a control. With the imagined pointing task, children with DCD did not conform to speed accuracy trade-offs during imagined movements, but all other groups did. However, on the hand rotation task, both the ADHD + DCD and DCD groups were less accurate than the ADHD and control groups. This study demonstrated that children with ADHD + DCD experience genuine motor control impairments manifested by a reduced ability to accurately represent movement – a problem that does not appear to be linked to increased levels of inattention or decreased working memory capacity typically observed in children with ADHD alone.

Motor imagery has also been recently explored with adults with probable DCD (Hyde et al., 2014). The authors found that while the performance profiles of young adults with pDCD indicated use of a MI strategy to complete a hand rotation task, they were nonetheless significantly less efficient when doing so. This finding demonstrates a similar pattern of impairment to that previously observed in children with DCD during hand rotation tasks.

While most studies have used the hand rotation task to explore MI capacity, one study has explored MI from a unique perspective in children with DCD. Caçola and colleagues (2014) used a combination of an estimation of reach paradigm that groups motor imagery with the extension of space via tool use. A tool is said to modify, at least temporally, the body schema, which is considered a functional element for perceiving one's own body in environmental space. In brief, tool use affords extension of the neural representation of ones's peripersonal (near) space, thus, tools may be important mediators between the body and our environment; a situation that presents challenge even to a young child. In TD children, research suggests that accuracy for arm and tool reach estimations are similar as early as 6 years of age (Caçola & Gabbard, 2012). A comparison between a TD and a DCD group of children indicated that compared to TD children, those with DCD have more difficulty estimating reach distances using the longer of two tool lengths: 40 cm compared to 20 cm. The authors concluded that this finding may be related to differences in quality of motor imagery and in the ability to create an effective internal model for action in this context. Furthermore, it was suggested that tool length may present an additional action processing constraint on children with DCD (Caçola et al., 2014).

In summary, the consistent pattern of MI deficit provides compelling evidence that children with DCD may experience difficulties engaging in MI. Based on the assumption that MI performance provides insight into the internal action representations that precede real movement, the bulk of the abovementioned studies have argued that the motor difficulties typical of DCD may arise, at least in part, from difficulties generating and/or implementing internal representations of movement.

Implications and Applications

Planning and prediction are fundamental for accurate motor behavior. Through motor imagery, it is possible to assess movement opportunities and foresee consequences before performing a motor skill. The understanding of the IMD hypothesis can provide significant insights into the screening and training of difficulties observed in patients with DCD. It has been noted that motor imagery training can cause improvements in speed, accuracy, and strength of motor execution (Lorey et al., 2010).

Motor imagery training has also been well studied in sports and is effective at improving players' performance and the acquisition of new skills (Atienza, Balaguer, & Garcia-Merita, 1998; Roure et al., 1999). However, motor imagery may be a more essential part of motor skill training in rehabilitation settings, as in many cases, motor function may not be present and motor imagery may be the only way to activate motor networks in the brain. In fact, in recent years, MI has emerged as a promising, noninvasive, and inexpensive technique to improve motor skill performance (Sun et al., 2013). MI has been proved to be an effective technique to assist in rehabilitation of motor function in several different conditions, including stroke, hemiplegia, and multiple sclerosis, to name a few (Lee et al., 2011; Schuster et al., 2012; Cho, Kim, & Lee, 2012).

More important, here, is the notion that motor imagery integrity may help educators and therapists diagnose and treat DCD. A pilot study (and the only one I am aware of) was conducted by Wilson et al. (2002) to determine whether a MI training protocol designed to improve children's ability to generate action representation was as effective as traditional perceptuo-motor training in facilitating skill development in children with poor motor skills. Fifty-four children participated in this study and were assigned to one of three groups: Imagery training, perceptual-motor training, and control. The motor imagery protocol involved the observation of video-audio sequences of a selection of fundamental motor skills (catching, throwing, striking, etc). Children then imagined performing each step of the skill, moving their body to each of the positions. Next, they observed videotapes of other children successfully performing the skills. Children were asked to create an action replay of the model, and then to imagine themselves performing the skill from external and internal perspectives. After this MI training, children engaged in several trials involving physical practice and mental rehearsal between skill attempts. The results indicated that the imagery protocol was shown to be equally effective to perceptual-motor training in facilitating the development of motor skills.

The authors state that the most remarkable finding of the study was that a protocol largely based on mental training can achieve the same effects as a traditional perceptual-motor training program (Wilson et al., 2002). According to them, the protocol was useful because they helped children develop a true motor/kinesthetic representation of an intended action. The sequence of steps involved in the protocol allowed children to shape their understanding of the skill and to develop a feel for the movement before overt practice occurs. The training of the “map” and “steps” to accomplish the correct form of a real motor skill may be shaping the motor parameters that determine how those skills unfold (Wilson et al., 2002).

Perhaps the most interesting aspect of MI is the fact that it can be used at home, unsupervised (or with parental supervision), and it is easier and more convenient to apply than traditional physical therapy methods. There is also great potential in adding a MI training component to conventional forms of intervention to see whether any gains can be further enhanced. In fact, most of the research conducted with MI training has demonstrated that the best use of MI is when combined with physical practice. Further research needs to be done with children with Developmental Coordination Disorder to determine the most appropriate frequency and intensity of motor imagery training added to a physical therapy protocol. Because of its ease and convenience, the more motor imagery added to a protocol, the better.

Other important considerations prior to beginning imagery training are to establish whether or not children can perform motor imagery (in the DCD case, this might be a very important factor) and what tasks are more suitable to the age and motor difficulties of the child. Finally, it is important to consider how the MI task interacts with and facilitates other activities that are included in the training/rehabilitation protocol. In physical therapy settings, motor imagery can be especially used for strength paradigms. For example, Lebon et al (2010) has suggested that individuals benefit from performing imagined muscle contractions, especially during rest periods of their physical training.

In addition, MI can be used any time that children with DCD have to analyze task demands, interpret environmental cues, use knowledge of performance for anticipatory preparation of their body, detect errors, and to correct movements. In fact, a cognitive perspective has been proven to be extremely beneficial in facilitating skill acquisition for DCD in occupational therapy settings (Hyland & Polatajko, 2012). This approach, called Cognitive Orientation to (daily) Occupational Performance (CO-OP), uses cognitive strategies to approach individualized goals. CO-OP is a verbally-based, individualized approach focused on guiding children to learn and discover cognitive strategies to solve motor problems (Polatajko, Mandich, Missiuna, et al., 2001; Polatajko & Mandich, 2004). It aims to teach children to use self-talk and problem-solving strategies to solve performance problems. Through intervention, the CO-OP therapist guides the child in the learning of a global problem solving strategy and the discovery of domain specific cognitive strategies that improve motor performance.

More specifically, when using CO-OP the child is encouraged to form a mental model of how to attack a movement task; by generating a movement goal, planning its implementation, and reflecting on how their performance was or was not successful (goal, plan, do, check) (Mandich, Polatajko, Missiuna, & Miller). Even though this strategy is mainly used in Occupational Therapy settings, I believe it can be implemented in physical therapy protocols as well. In fact, the CO-OP method is a great way of implementing motor imagery in therapeutic settings. The "planning" of a goal may include how to perform the skill, and the therapist may focus on MI at this stage, as well as in the "checking" stage, with MI being used to explore whether the action was performed correctly, and if not, how to do so.

In summary, motor imagery training can be used to improve motor skills of children with DCD. I believe that MI can be easily added into any rehabilitation protocol along with physical practice.

Conclusion

DCD is a motor skill disorder that negatively affects a child's ability to perform everyday tasks. In this chapter, I provided evidence that children with DCD have an underlying deficit in generating and/or monitoring internal models of action, the so-called IMD hypothesis. This hypothesis has been largely accepted as one of the likely causes of the motor skill difficulties presented in DCD. Because of that, use of motor imagery training should be considered in rehabilitation settings. This cognitive approach may not intuitive to physical therapists, but might provide improvement of motor skills if added to rehabilitation protocols, as confirmed by studies with other conditions and one study that proved its efficacy with children with DCD. In summary, I recommend that components of motor imagery training be added to physical therapy settings, in addition to physical training.

References

Adams, I. L. J., Lust, J. M., Wilson, P. H., & Steenbergen, B. (2014). Compromised motor control in children with DCD: A deficit in the internal model? A systematic review. *Neuroscience and Biobehavioral Reviews, 47,* 225-244. doi:10.1016/j.neubiorev.2014.08.011.

American Psychiatric Association (2013). *Diagnostic and statistical manual of mental disorders* (5th ed.). Washington: American Psychiatric Association.

Atienza, F. L., Balaguer, I., Garcia-Merita, M. L. (1998). Video modeling and imaging training on performance of tennis service of 9- to 12-year-old children. *Perceptual Motor Skills, 87,* 519–529.

Butson, M. L., Hyde, C., Steenbergen, B., & Williams, J. (2014). Assessing motor imagery using the hand rotation task: does performance change across childhood? *Human Movement Science, 35,* 50–65.

Bo, J., & Lee, C. M. (2013). Motor skill learning in children with Developmental Coordination Disorder. *Research in Developmental Disabilities, 34,* 2047-2055. doi: 10.1016/j.ridd.2013.03.012

Caçola, P. (2014). Movement difficulties affect children's learning: An overview of Developmental Coordination Disorder (DCD). *Learning Disabilities: A Multidisciplinary Journal, 20*(2), 98-106.

Caçola, P. & Gabbard, C. (2012). Modulating peripersonal and extrapersonal reach space: A developmental perspective. *Experimental Brain Research, 218*(2), 321-330. doi: 10.1007/s00221-012-3017-8

Caçola, P., Gabbard, C., Ibana, M., & Romero, M. (2014). Tool length influences reach distance estimation via motor imagery in children with Developmental Coordination Disorder. *Journal of Clinical and Experimental Neuropsychology, 36*(6), 596-606. doi: 10.1080/13803395.2014.918092

Cairney, J., Hay, J., Faught, B., & Hawes, R. (2005). Developmental Coordination Disorder and overweight and obesity in children aged 9–14 years. *International Journal of Obesity, 29*(4), 369–372.

Campbell, W. N., Missiuna, C., & Vaillancourt, T. (2012). Peer victimization and depression in children with and without motor coordination difficulties. *Psychology in the Schools, 49*(4), 328-341.

Caeyenberghs, K., Tsoupas, J., Wilson, P. H., & Smits-Engelsman, B. C. M. (2009). Motor imagery in primary school children. *Developmental Neuropsychology, 34*(1), 103–121. doi: 10.1080/87565640802499183

Cho, H., Kim, J., & Lee, G. (2012). Effects of motor imagery training on balance and gait abilities in post-stroke patients: A randomized controlled trial. *Clinical Rehabilitation, 27*(8), 675-680.

Decety, J., & Grezes, J. (1999). Neural mechanisms subserving the perception of human actions. *Trends in Cognitive Sciences, 3*, 172-178.

Deconinck, F. J. A., Spitaels, L., Fias, W., & Lenoir, M. (2009). Is Developmental Coordination Disorder a motor imagery deficit? *Journal of Clinical and Experimental Neuropsychology, 31*, 720–730. doi: 10.1080/13803390802484805.

Funk, M., Brugger, P., & Wilkening, F. (2005). Motor processes in children's imagery: The case of mental rotation of hands. *Developmental Science, 8*(5), 402-408.

Gabbard, C. (2009). Studying action representation in children via motor imagery. *Brain and Cognition, 71*, 234-239.

Gabbard, C., & Bobbio, T. (2011). The inability to mentally represent action may be associated with performance deficits in children with Developmental Coordination Disorder. *International Journal of Neuroscience, 121*(3), 113-120. doi: 10.3109/00207454.2010.535936

Gabbard, C., Caçola, P., & Lee, J. (2013). *The role of motor imagery in action planning: Implications for developmental research.* In M. L. & M. F. (Eds.), Motor Behavior and Control: New Research, Volume xx, (pp. 23-40). Nova Science Publishers, Inc.

Gibbs, J., Appleton, J., & Appleton, R. (2007). Dyspraxia or Developmental Coordination Disorder? Unravelling the enigma. *Archives of Disease in Childhood, 92*(6), 534–539.

Green, D., Baird, G., & Sugden, D. (2006). A pilot study of psychopathology in developmental coordination disorder. *Child: Care, Health, and Development, 32*, 741-50.

Henderson, S. E., & Henderson, L. (2002). Toward an understanding of Developmental Coordination Disorder. *Adapted Physical Activity Quarterly, 19*(1), 11–31.

Hyde, C., Fuelscher, I., Buckthought, K., Enticott, P. G., Gitay, M. A., & Williams, J. (2014). Motor imagery is less efficient in adults with probable Developmental Coordination Disorder: Evidence from the hand rotation task. *Research in Developmental Disabilities, 35*, 3062-3070. doi:10.1016/j.ridd.2014.07.042.

Hyde, C., & Wilson, P. (2011a). Online motor control in children with Developmental Coordination Disorder: chronometric analysis of double-step reaching performance. *Child: Care, Health, and Development, 37*(1), 111–122. doi: 10.1111/j.1365-2214.2010.01131.x.

Hyde, C., & Wilson, P.H. (2011b). Dissecting online control in Developmental Coordination Disorder: a kinematic analysis of double-step reaching. B*rain & Cognition, 75*(3), 232–241. doi:10.1016/ j.bandc.2010.12.004.

Holsti, L., Grunau, R. V., & Whitfield, M. F. (2002). Developmental Coordination Disorder in extremely low birth weight children at nine years. *Journal of Developmental and Behavioral Pediatrics, 23*(1), 9–15.

Hyland, M., & Polatajko, H. J. (2012). Enabling children with Developmental Coordination Disorder to self-regulate through the use of Dynamic Performance Analysis: Evidence from the CO-OP approach. *Human Movement Science, 31*(4), 987-998. doi:10.1016/j.humov.2011.09.003.

Isaac, A. R., Marks, D. F. & Russell, D. G. (1986). An instrument for assessing imagery of movement: The Vividness of Movement Imagery Questionnaire (VMIQ). *Journal of Mental Imagery, 10*(4), 1986, 23–30.

Jeannerod, M. (2001). Neural simulation of action: A unifying mechanism for motor cognition. *Neuroimage, 14*, 103–109.

Jover, M., Schmitz, C., Centelles, L., Chabrol, B., & Assaiante, C. (2010). Anticipatory postural adjustments in a bimanual load-lifting task in children with Developmental Coordination Disorder. *Developmental Medicine & Child Neurology, 52*(9), 850-855. doi:10.1111/j.1469-8749.2009.03611.x.

Jucaite, A., Fernell, E., Forssberg, H., & Hadders-Algra, M. (2003). Deficient coordination of associated postural adjustments during a lifting task in children with neurodevelopmental disorders. *Developmental Medicine & Child Neurology, 45*(11), 731–742.

Langaas, T., Mon-Williams, M., Wann, J.P., Pascal, E., & Thompson, C. (1998). Eye movements, prematurity and Developmental Co-Ordination Disorder. *Vision Research, 38*(12), 1817–1826. doi:S0042698997003994.

Lebon, F, Collet, C, & Guillot, A. (2010). Benefits of motor imagery training on muscle strength. *Journal of Strength & Conditioning Research,* 24(6), 1680-1687.

Lee, G., Song, C., Lee, Y., Cho, H., & Lee, S. (2011). Effects of motor imagery training on gait ability of patients with chronic stroke. *Journal of Physical Therapy Science, 23*, 197-200.

Lewis, M., Vance, A., Maruff, P., Wilson, P., & Cairney, S. (2008). Differences in motor imagery between children with developmental coordination disorder with and without the combined type of ADHD. *Developmental Medicine & Child Neurology, 50*(8), 608–612. doi: 10.1111/j.1469-8749.2008.03030.x

Lorey, B., Pilgramm, S., Walter, B., Stark, R., Munzert, J., Zentgraf, K. (2010). Your mind's hand: Motor imagery of pointing movements with different accuracy. *NeuroImage, 49*(4), 3239-3247.

Katschmarsky, S., Cairney, S., Maruff, P., Wilson, P.H., & Currie, J. (2001). The ability to execute saccades on the basis of efference copy: impairments in double-step saccade performance in children with developmental co-ordination disorder. *Experimental Brain Research, 136*(1), 73–78.

Mackenzie, S. J., Getchell, N., Deutsch, K., Wilms-Floet, A., Clark, J. E., & Whitall, J. (2008). Multi-limb coordination and rhythmic variability under varying sensory availability conditions in children with DCD. *Human Movement Science, 27*(2), 256–269.

Malouin, F., Richards, C. L., & Durand, A. (2010). Normal aging and motor imagery vividness: Implications for mental practice training in rehabilitation. *Archives of Physical Medicine and Rehabilitation, 91*(7), 1122–1127.

Mandich, A., Polatajko, H., Missiuna, C., Miller, L. (2001). Cognitive strategies and motor performance in children with Developmental Coordination Disorder. *Physical and Occupational Therapy in Pediatrics, 20*, 125–143.

Maruff, P., Wilson, P., Trebilcock, M., & Currie, J. (1999) Abnormalities of imagined motor sequences in children with Developmental Coordination Disorder. *Neuropsychologia, 37*, 1317-1324.

Missiuna, C., Rivard, L., & Pollock, N. (2004). They're bright but can't write: Developmental Coordination Disorder in school-aged children. *Teaching Exceptional Children Plus, 1*(1), 3.

Molina, M., Tijus, C., & Jouen, F. (2008). The emergence of motor imagery in children. *Journal of Experimental Child Psychology, 99*(3), 196-209.

Munzert, J., Lorey, B., & Zentgraf, K. (2009). Cognitive motor processes: The role of motor imagery in the study of motor representations. *Brain Research Reviews, 60*(2), 306–326.

Noten, M., Wilson, P., Ruddock, S., & Steenbergen, B. (2014). Mild impairments of motor imagery skills in children with DCD. *Research in Developmental Disabilities, 35*(5), 1152–1159.

Pereira, H. S., Landgren, M., Gillberg, C., & Forssberg, H. (2001). Parametric control of fingertip forces during precision grip lifts in children with DCD (developmental coordination disorder) and DAMP (deficits in attention motor control and perception). *Neuropsychologia, 39*(5), 478–488. doi:S0028-3932(00)00132-9.

Pettit, L., Charles, J., Wilson, A. D., Plumb, M. S., Brockman, A., Williams, J. H. G., & Williams, M. (2008). Constrained action selection in children with developmental coordination disorder. *Human Movement Science, 27*(2), 286–295. doi: 10.1016/j.humov.2008.02.014

Polatajko, H. J., & Cantin, N. (2005). *Developmental Coordination Disorder (dyspraxia): An overview of the state of the art.* Paper presented at the Seminars in Pediatric Neurology. Polatajko, H. J., Mandich, A. D., Miller, L.T., & Macnab, J. J. (2001). Cognitive Orientation to daily Occupational Performance (CO-OP): Part 2 – The evidence. *Physical and Occupational Therapy in Pediatrics, 20*, 83–106.

Polatajko, H. J., & Mandich, A. (2004). Enabling occupation in children: The Cognitive Orientation to daily Occupational Performance (CO-OP) approach. (1st ed.). CAOT Publications ACE, Ottawa, ON.

Roure, R., Collet, C., Deschaumes-Molinaro, C., et al. (1999). Imagery quality estimated by autonomic response is correlated to sporting performance enhancement. *Physiology & Behavior, 66*, 63–72.

Steenbergen, B., Van Nimwegen, M., Crajé, C. (2007). Solving a mental rotation task in congenital hemiparesis: Motor imagery versus visual imagery. *Neuropsychologia, 45*(14), 3324–3328.

Schuster, C., Butler, J., Andrews, B., Kischka, U., & Ettlin, T. (2012). Comparison of embedded and added motor imagery training in patients after stroke: Results of a randomized controlled pilot trial. *Trials, 13*, 11.

Tsai, C., Pan, C., Cherng, R., Hsu, Y., Chiu, H. (2009). Mechanisms of deficit of visuo-spatial attention shift in children with Developmental Coordination Disorder: A neurophysiological measure of the endogenous Posner paradigm. *Brain and Cognition, 71*, 246–258.

Toussaint, L., Tahej, P. K., Thibaut, J. P., Possamai, C. A., & Badets, A. (2013). On the link between action planning and motor imagery: a developmental study. *Experimental Brain Research, 231*(3), 331–339.

VanWaelvelde, H., deWeerdt, W., de Cock, P., Janssens, L., Feys, H., & Bouwien, C. M. (2006). Parameterization of movement execution in children with developmental coordination disorder. *Brain and Cognition, 60*(1), 20–31. doi: 10.1016/j.bandc.2005.08.004

Williams, J., Omizzolo, C., Galea, M., & Vance, A. (2013). Motor imagery skills of children with Attention Deficit Hyperactivity Disorder and Developmental Coordination Disorder. *Human Movement Science, 32*, 121-135. doi: 10.1016/j.humov.2012.08.003

Williams, J., Thomas, P. R., Maruff, P., Butson, M., & Wilson, P. H. (2006). Motor, visual and egocentric transformations in children with Developmental Coordination Disorder. *Child: Care, Health and Development, 32*, 633–647. doi: 10.1111/j.1365-2214.2006.00688.x

Williams, J., Thomas, P. R., Maruff, P., & Wilson, P. H. (2008). The link between motor impairment level and motor imagery ability in children with Developmental Coordination Disorder. *Human Movement Science, 27*, 270–285. doi: 10.1016/j.humov.2008.02.008

Wilmut, K., Brown, J. H., & Wann, J. P. (2007). Attention disengagement in children with Developmental Coordination Disorder. *Disability and Rehabilitation, 29* (1), 47- 55. doi:10.1080/09638280600947765.

Wilson, P. H., & Maruff, P. (1999). Deficits in the endogenous control of covert visuospatial attention in children with Developmental Coordination Disorder. Human Movement Science, 18 (2–3), 421–442. doi: 10.1016/S0167-9457(99)00017-2.

Wilson, P.H., Maruff, P., McKenzie, B.E. (1997). Covert orienting of visuospatial attention in children with Developmental Coordination Disorder. *Developmental Medicine & Child Neurology, 39*(11), 736–745.

Wilson, P. H., Maruff, P., Butson, M., Williams, J., Lum, J., & Thomas, P. R. (2004). Internal representation of movement in children with Developmental Coordination Disorder: A mental rotation task. *Developmental Medicine & Child Neurology, 46*, 754–759. doi: 10.1017/S001216220400129X

Wilson, P. H., Ruddock, S., Smits-Engelsman, B., Polatajko, H., & Blank, R. (2013). Understanding performance deficits in Developmental Coordination Disorder: A meta-analysis of recent research. *Developmental Medicine & Child Neurology, 55*, 217-228. doi: 10.1111/j.1469-8749.2012.04436.x

Wilson, P. H., Thomas, P. R., & Maruff, P. (2002). Motor imagery training ameliorates motor clumsiness in children. Journal of Child Neurology, 17(7), 491-498.

Wolpert, D. M. (1997). Computational approaches to motor control. *Trends in Cognitive Sciences, 1*, 209–216.

Zoia, S., Barnett, A., Wilson, P., & Hill, E. (2006). Developmental Coordination Disorder: Current issues. *Child: Care, health, and development, 32*, 613-618. doi: 10.1111/j.1365-2214.2006.00697.x

Zwicker, J. G., Missiuna, C., Harris, S. R., Boyd, L. A. (2012). Developmental Coordination Disorder: A review and update. *European Journal of Paediatric Neurology, 16*(6), 573-581. doi:10.1016/j.ejpn.2012.05.005

In: Motor Imagery
Editor: Brandon M. Garcia

ISBN: 978-1-63483-125-3

Chapter 3

The Potential of Motor Imagery Training in Fall Prevention among the Elderly

Carl Gabbard [*]
Texas A&M University, Texas, US

Abstract

Contemporary research findings indicate that in older persons (typically 64 > years) there are functional decrements in the ability to mentally represent and effectively plan motor actions. That is, many older persons do not effectively simulate (via mental imagery) prior actions resulting in intentions that are significantly different from movement execution. For example, our work and others have reported that, compared to younger adults, older persons typically show greater over- or underestimation of abilities, such as when reaching and stepping. Such incorrections may, especially with the elderly, lead to loss of postural control (balance) and a higher risk of falling. This chapter: (1) highlights research findings on mental representation and motor imagery in the elderly, (2) describes the effectiveness and potential of motor imagery training in general, (3) addresses the implications for improving

[*] Corresponding author: Carl Gabbard, Professor, TAMU 4243, College Station TX 77843; 979.845.1277.

movement efficiency and lowering the risk of movement-related injury, and finally, (4) provides guidelines / strategies for motor imagery practice in the context of reach planning.

Introduction

Recent research findings indicate that with older adulthood (approximately 64 years >), there are functional decrements in spatial cognition and more specially, in the ability to mentally represent and effectively plan motor actions. That is, many older persons do not effectively simulate (via mental imagery) prior actions resulting in intentions that are significantly different from movement execution. A typical finding is a significant over- or underestimation of one's actual physical abilities with movement planning—planning that has implications for movement efficiency and physical safety. A practical, daily life example is estimation of reachability—a situation that for the elderly may be linked with fall incidence. A strategy used to mentally represent action is the use of motor imagery— an ability that also declines with advancing older age.

This chapter begins with a discussion of research findings on mental representation and motor imagery ability in the elderly. Next, it describes the effectiveness and potential of motor imagery training in general, then I address the implications for using motor imagery practice to improve movement efficiency and lower the risk of movement-related injury. And finally, the chapter concludes by providing guidelines / strategies for creating a motor imagery program in the context of reach planning.

Mentally Representing Action and Motor Imagery

Motor programming theory proposes that internal (*forward*) models make predictions (*estimates*) by mapping the self to parameters of the external world to enable successful planning and execution of action. An internal model is a neural system that simulates the dynamic behavior (movement) of the body in relation to the environment (e.g., Wolpert, 1997). An adequate internal model -- *action representation* of a movement -- is required for an effective outcome. In typical conditions, internal models are continuously updated on the basis of experience. Motor imagery, also known as kinesthetic imagery, is an active cognitive process during which the representation of a specific action is internally reproduced in working memory without any overt motor output (Decety & Grezes, 1999). *Motor imagery provides a window into the process of action representation by reflecting an internal action representation* (Chabeauti et al., 2012; Jeannerod, 2001; Munzert et al., 2009; Wintermute, 2012). The theory that motor control and motor simulation states are functionally equivalent (Kraeutner et al., 2014; Kunz et al., 2009; Lorey et al., 2009) postulates that mental (covert) and executed (overt) actions rely on similar motor representations (Pelgrims et al., 2009). Studies have found a high correlation between real and simulated movements (e.g., Heremans et al., 2007; Sharma et al., 2008; Young et al., 2009). In action planning, the ability to predict an intended action's outcome and consequences is important. It has also been hypothesized that motor imagery plays an important role in predicting actions (e.g., Bourgeois & Coello, 2009; Kunz et al., 2009; Lorey et al., 2009; Springer et al., 2012): for example, when planning an intended action, using imagery to consider important timing and biomechanical information helps predict the movement's sensory consequences. Suddendorf and Moore (2011) note, "The ability to imagine future events is an essential part of human cognition" (p. 295). Imagery allows us to generate specific predictions based upon past experience and allows us to answer 'what if' questions by making explicit and accessible the likely consequences of a specific action. Imagining an action can serve several useful goals to that endeavor.

Motor Imagery Ability in Older Persons

Recent observations indicate that the ability to mentally represent motor actions declines with advancing age (> 64 years; Beauchet et al., 2010; Caçola et al., 2013; Mulder et al., 2008; Personnier et al., 2010; Saimpont et al., 2010; Skoura et al., 2008; Zapparoli et al., 2013). For example, using a mental chronometry paradigm with imagined and executed arm pointing action in young and older adults, Personnier and colleagues found that although the older adults used efferent copies of motor commands to generate motor representations (i.e., they displayed the ability to mentally represent action), this ability progressively deteriorated with advancing age as evidenced by the declining quality of their motor imagery (i.e., isochrony between executed and imagined movements). These findings also indicate the likelihood of weakness in the formulation of internal models of action in the elderly.

Research findings provide evidence of older adults' declining ability to mentally represent action. Examining the relation between vividness of movement imagery via questionnaire, Mulder and colleagues (2008) found that older adults were slightly worse than their younger counterparts, especially from a first person perspective. A possible link between level of physical activity and imagery ability was suggested but not tested. Testing the ability to mentally simulate/plan a complex sequential action of the whole body (i.e., rising from the floor), Saimpont et al. (2010) reported the elderly experienced significant difficulties compared to young adults' accuracy in action sequence and reaction time. In a more recent review of this body of research pertaining to individuals 55 years and older, Saimpont and colleagues (2013) concluded that motor imagery accuracy for simple / usual upper-limb movements appears well preserved with aging whereas there appears to be an aging effect with upper-limb actions with unusual biomechanical constraints.

To summarize, it would appear that older persons have difficulty estimating possible movement outcomes and updating internal models, resulting in a dissociation between perception and action; a condition that may promote risky motor planning.

Reach Planning and Its Implications

Since our focus on the potential of motor imagery practice is with reach planning, a brief background is warranted. Estimation of whether an object is reachable or not from a specific body position constitutes an important aspect in effective motor planning; a situation that has both scientific and real-world implications. That estimation is based in large part on the individual's ability to mentally represent the desired action and a function of perceived body capabilities. An experimental tactic that provides insight into this phase of motor planning (estimation) is estimation of reach via use of motor imagery. That methodology has drawn the interest of contemporary researchers for examining the processes involved in action representation (Coello et al., 2008; Lamm et al., 2007). Estimation of reach complements the internal modeling notion of "can I do this?" and, "what are the consequences?" which arguably, are relevant questions in planning movements. More specific to reach, one of the initial steps in programming such movements is to derive a perceptual estimate of the object's distance and location relative to the body. This means that an individual must be able to perceive critical reach distances beyond which a particular reach action is no longer afforded and to which a transition to another reach mode must occur. For example, is the object close enough to reach while seated, or do I need to stand? Furthermore, with older persons, could I lose balance and fall? Such questions are not uncommon in every day situations, for example: reaching for an object on a table or reaching and grasping a hand rail.

More in line with the 'reaching' context used as an example in the chapter, research has found that overestimation of action capabilities in the context of reaching is a common observation among older adults (e.g., Gabbard et al., 2011; Noël et al., 2011). Gabbard and colleagues reported that younger adults (mean age 20 years) were significantly more accurate than older adults (mean age 77 years) when estimating reach in peripersonal and extrapersonal space from a seating position. Whereas both groups made more errors in extrapersonal space, the values were significantly higher for the older group; that is, they overestimated to a greater extent. In 2012, Caçola and colleagues reported that accuracy decreased as age increased when estimating reachability in peripersonal and extrapersonal space using a 40 cm tool; the population ranged from 55- to 92 years. To summarize, it would appear that older persons have difficulty estimating possible movement outcomes and updating internal models, resulting in a dissociation between perception and action; a condition that may promote risky motor planning. These studies and a review by Gabbard and Fox (2013) suggest thtat overestimation of actions could be a contributing factor in fall risk.

One example of daily living 'actual' reach with implications for physical safety is functional reach. Commonly used when assessing the elderly, functional reach is the maximal distance an individual is capable of reaching forward while standing, without taking a step or losing balance. It is described as a dynamic measure of postural control. The literature supports the observation that with advancing age there is a sharp decline in functional reach (Costarella et al., 2010; Zuccaro et al., 2012). And, perhaps most relevant to considerations of safety, research also indicates a significant relationship between functional reach and risk of falling (Duncan et al., 1990; Huang et al., 2003). In a recent study of young adults (mean age 22 years) and older adults (66 years) examining the relationship between estimation of reach and functional reach, Gabbard and Cordova (2013) reported that only the younger group showed a significant association between the two variables. In other words, the congruence between movement planning (estimation) and execution was significantly better with the younger group.

In regard to injury risk is the higher likelihood, compared to younger adults, of falling during reach actions. For example, if an older adult either significantly underestimates or overestimates a reach target (e.g., drinking glass, table, railing), they may have more difficulty than a younger person in maintaining postural control resulting in a fall. According to a view of the latest CDC website, "Each year, one in every three adults age 65 and older falls." "Among older adults (those 65 or older), falls are the leading cause of injury death." In partial support of the reach – fall link, four of 16 items on the Activities-Specific Balance Confidence (ABC) Scale (Powell & Myers, 1995), are reach specific questions. That test is commonly cited as a self-report subjective measure of perceived balance confidence in performing various movement activities without falling. As noted earlier, whereas the cause of falling in older persons is multifaceted (e.g., disease, medications, visual impairment, balance, environmental factors), recent findings suggest that one of the underlying problems is difficulty in mentally representing and planning intended movements (e.g., Caçola et al., 2013; Paizis et al., 2014; Zapparoli et al., 2013). Furthermore, another review study that looked at the circumstances of falls in elderly people, reported that incorrect transfer or shift of bodyweight was the most frequent cause of falling (41%) (Robinovitch et al., 2013). A specific example was leaning too far from one's base of support; an observation commonly seen during overestimation in reach situations.

Motor Imagery Practice

One, if not the most evident finding associated with motor imagery, is its potential as a therapeutic tool. Use of motor imagery has been documented as an effective training and therapy tool for: sport / motor performance (Gentili et al., 2010; Guillot et al., 2010; Zhang et al., 2011; Lebon et al., 2010), brain injury (Osstra et al., 2012), stroke (Cho et al., 2012; Hosseini et al., 2012; see reviews by Malouin & Richards, 2010; Sharma et al., 2009), and other neuromotor impairments (Heremans et al., 2012). For motor performance, studies commonly suggest that imagery training facilitates motor learning processes and improves motor performance. In the context of neurological impairment, the literature suggests that one of the key agents in movement recovery is use of motor imagery to stimulate otherwise non-active or impaired neural pathways. In addition, Wohldmann and colleagues (2008) reported evidence to support the hypothesis that mental practice strengthens abstract mental representation that does not involve specific effectors. That is, such practice strengthens 'central' features of the representation as well as representation of specific body part processes. To examine the hypothesis, the researchers had participants type 4-digit numbers in a familiarization phase, training phase (using imagined and actual execution with a different digit configuration or the opposite hand), and delay condition (actual execution using same setup as the familiarization); the fingers represented specific movement effectors. It is also important to note that of either visual or motor (kinesthetic) imagery, motor imagery, as proposed here, has shown to be more effective in cortiomotor stimulation (e.g., Guillot et al., 2004; Stinear et al., 2006; Voisin et al., 2011).

General Strategies for Motor Imagery Practice

Whereas the information on clinical strategies to improve mental imagery among the elderly is sparse, information derived from training studies among brain and stroke patients may be applicable (e.g., Langhome et al., 2009; Schuster et al., 2011). Those strategies include (as suggested by Gabbard & Fox, 2013):

- *Clear and effective script of instructions:* The script of instructions should be used in early practice phases and needs to be as specific as possible. For example: "Watch and feel your hand and fingers reaching and grasping the mug. How will you grasp the mug and how fast will you move as not to spill its contents?"
- *Goal-setting:* This is an important element of practice and a strategy that can be induced via the script, verbally, or in combination as reinforcement.
- *First person internalizing:* That is, focus on the self as the mental image of the intended action. This state is the first component in the actor-object dyad. Part of this dyad is an understanding of one's physical capabilities and potential consequences. Ask the participant to consider the consequences if he or she were to miss-plan (over- or underestimate) the event. What will you fall into? Do you feel confident in your ability to gain stability if you have to adjust your position quickly?

- *Concentrate on the effectors:* This is the specific part of the self that is linked with the target. For example, focus on the arm/hand when intending to reach and grasp an object.
- *Focus on the visual cues (target/object/goal):* Concentrate on the end point of the intended action–the target. For example, where does my hand need to be to grasp the object securely? With tasks such as aiming at a target, when timing is a factor, auditory cues in the form of a metronome have been effective.
- *Reinforcement on kinesthetically 'feeling' execution of movement:* Research indicates clearly that 'feeling' rather than just seeing oneself perform the action promotes better mental representation for movement via internalization.
- *Combine physical practice with mental practice:* By practicing actual movements, participants gain a better understanding of their physical capabilities and develop movement endurance, a problem that is common in the elderly. Physical practice affords the opportunity to test one's capabilities. Furthermore, research shows that mental practice combined with physical practice enhances actual performance outcome (Schuster et al., 2011; Reiser et al., 2011).
- *Progress from simple to more complex actions:* Do this when practicing both imagined and actual execution movements.
- *Practice 15-60 minutes, 3 times/week for 4 weeks:* This has been one of the most commonly reported practice durations with a variety of patient impairments. Obviously, this should be viewed as an approximate benchmark with the progression principle strictly applied.

Conclusion

Research findings present a relatively clear indication that with the elderly, the ability to effectively plan intended actions becomes increasingly more difficult. As in the context of reach, that ineffectiveness could present a higher risk of falling. Given that imagery training, specifically motor imagery training, has been effective in improving motor behavior with different populations, this chapter has shown that imagery training may be useful in reducing fall risk in the elderly.

References

Beauchet, O., Annweiler, C., Assal, F., Bridenbaugh, S., Hermann, R. R., Kressig, R. W., & Allali, G. (2010). Imagined Timed Up & Go test: A new tool to assess higher- level gait and balance disorders in older adults? *Journal of Neurological Sciences, 294*(1), 102-106.

Bourgeois, J., & Coello, Y. (2009). Role of inertial properties of the upper limb on the perception of the boundary of personal space. *Psychologie Française*, *54*(3), 225- 239.

Caçola, P., Martinez, A., & Ray, C. (2012). The ability to modulate peripersonal and extrapersonal *reach space via tool use among the elderly. Archives of Gerontology and Geriatrics, 56*(2), 383–388.

Caçola, P., Roberson, J., & Gabbard, C. (2013). Aging in movement representations for sequential finger movements: A comparison between young, middle-aged, and older adults. *Brain and Cognition*, *82*(1), 1-5.

Chabeauti, P.Y., Assaiante, C., & Vaugoyeau, M. (2012). Extreme short-term environmental constraints do not update internal models of action as assessed from motor imagery in adults. *Neuroscience, 222, 69-74.*

Cho, H.Y., Kim, J.S., & Lee, G.C. (2012). Effects of motor imagery training on balance and gait abilities in post-stroke patients: a randomized controlled trial. *Clinical Rehabilitation, 27(*8), 675-678.

Coello, Y., Bartolo, A., Amiri, B., Devanne, H., Houdayer, E., & Derambure, P. (2008). Perceiving what is reachable depends on motor representations: Evidence from transcranial magnetic stimulation study. *PLoS ONE, 3*(8), e2862.

Costarella, M., Monteleone, L., Steindler, R., & Zuccaro, S. M. (2010). Decline of physical and cognitive conditions in the elderly measured through the functional reach test and the mini-mental state examination. *Archives of Gerontology and Geriatrics, 50*(3), 332-337.

Decety, J., & Grezes, J. (1999). Neural mechanisms subserving the perception of human actions. *Trends in Cognitive Sciences, 3*, 172-178.

Duncan, P. W., Weiner, D. K., Chandler, J., & Studenski, S. (1990). Functional reach: a new clinical measure of balance. *Journal of Gerontology*, *45*(6), M192–M197.

Gabbard, C., Cacola, P., & Cordova, A. (2011). Is there an advanced aging effect on the ability to mentally represent action? *Archives of Geronology & Geriatrics*, *53*, 206–209.

Gabbard, C., & Cordova, A. (2013). Association between imagined and actual functional reach: A comparison of young and older adults. *Archives of Gerontology and Geriatrics. 56,* 487–491.

Gabbard, C. & Fox, A. (2013). Using motor imagery therapy to improve movement efficiency and reduce fall injury risk, *Journal of Novel Physiotherapies, 3*, 186-189.

Gentili, R., Han, C. E., Schweighofer, N., & Papaxanthis, C. (2010). Motor learning without doing: Trial-by-trial improvement in motor performance during mental training. *Journal of Neurophysiology, 104*(2), 774-783.

Guillot, A., Tolleron, C., & Collet, C. (2010). Does motor imagery enhance stretching and flexibility? *Journal of Sports Sciences, 28*(3), 291-298.

Heremans, E., Nieuwboer, A., Spildooren, J., De Bondt, S., D'Hooge, A. M., Helsen, W., & Feys, P. (2012). Cued motor imagery in patients with multiple sclerosis. *Neuroscience, 206*, 115–121,

Hosseini, S. A., Fallahpour, M., Syadi, M., Gharib, M., & Haghgoo, H. (2012). The impact of mental practice on stroke patient's postural balance. *Journal of the Neurological Sciences, 322*(1-2), 263–267.

Huang, H., Gau, M., Chuan, W., & Kernohan, G. (2003). Assessing risk of falling in older adults. *Public Health Nursing, 20*, 99–411.

Jeannerod, M. (2001). Neural simulation of action: a unifying mechanism for motor cognition. *Neuroimage, 14*, S103-109.

Kraeutner, S., Gionfriddo, A., Bardouille, T., & Boe, S. (2014). Motor imagery-based brain activity parallels that of motor execution: Evidence from magnetic source imagining of cortical oscillations. *Brain Research*, doi.org/10.1016/j.brainres.2014.09.001.

Kunz, B. R., Creem-Regehr, S. H., & Thompson, W.B. (2009). Evidence for motor simulation in imagined locomotion. *Journal of Experimental Psychology: Human Perception and Performance, 35*(5), 1458-1471.

Lamm, C., Fischer, M. H., & Decety, J. (2007). Predicting the actions of others taps into one's own somatosensory representations – A functional MRI study. *Neuropsychologia, 45*, 2480–2491.

Langhome, P, Coupar, F., & Pollock, A. (2009). Motor recovery after stroke: A systematic review. *Lancet Neurology, 8*, 741–54.

Lebon, F., Collet, C., & Guillot, A. (2010). Benefits of motor imagery training on muscle strength. *Journal of Strength and Conditioning Research*, 24(6), 1680-1687.

Lorey, B., Bischoff, M., Pilgramm, S., Stark, R., Munzert, J., & Zentgraf, K. (2009). The embodied nature of motor imagery: The influence of posture and perspective. *Experimental Brain Research, 194*, 233-243.

Malouin, F., & Richards, C. L. (2010). Mental practice for relearning locomotor skills. *Physical Therapy, 90*(2), 240-251.

Mulder, T., Hochstenbach, J. B. H., Heuvelena, M. J. G., & Otter, A. R. (2008). Motor imagery: The relation between age and imagery capacity. *Human Movement Science, 26*(2), 203–211.

Munzert, J., Lorey, B., & Zentgraf, K. (2009). Cognitive motor processes: The role of motor imagery in the study of motor representations. *Brain Research Reviews*, *60*(2), 306-326.

Noël, Bernard, & Luyat, (2011). The overestimation of performance: a specific bias of aging? Geriatric Psychology and Neuropsychiatrics Vieil, *9*(3), 287-294.

Osstra, K. M., Vereecke, A., Jones, K., Vanderstraeten, G., & Vingerhoets, G. (2012). Motor imagery ability in patients with tramatic brain injury. *Archives of Physical Medicine and Rehabilitation, 93*(5), 828-833.

Personnier, P., Bally, Y., & Papaxanthis, C. (2010). Mentally represented motor actions in normal aging III: Electromyographic features of imagined arm movements. *Behavioural Brain Research, 206,* 184–190.

Pelgrims, B., Andres, M., & Olivier, E. (2005). Motor imagery while judging object- hand interactions. *NeuroReport, 16*(11), 1193-1196.

Paizis, C., Skoura, X., Personnier, P., & Papaxanthis, C. (2014). Motor asymmetry attenuation in older adults during imagined arm movements. *Frontiers in Aging Neuroscience, 6,* 49.

Powell, L. E., & Myers, A. M. (1995). The activities-specific balance confidence (ABC) scale. *Journal of Gerontology A: Biological Science Medical Science, 50A (1),* M28–M34.

Reiser, M., Busch, D., & Munzert, J. (2011). Strength gains by motor imagery with different ratios of physical to mental practice. *Frontiers in Psychology, 2*, 194.

Robinovich, S., Feldman, F., Yang, Y., Schonnop, R., Leung, P. M., Sarraf, T.,..... Loughlin, M. (2013). Video capture of the circumstances of falls in elderly people residing in long-term care: An observational study. *Lancet, 381*, 47-54.

Saimpont, A., Malouin, F., Tousignant, B., & Jackson, P. (2013). Motor imagery and aging. *Journal of Motor Behavior, 45*(1), 21-28.

Saimpont A, Mourey F, Manckoundia P, Pfitzenmeyer P, & Pozzo T. (2010). Aging affects the mental simulation / planning of the ''rising from the floor'' sequence. *Archives in Gerontology and Geriatrics*, *51*, 41–e45.

Schuster, C., Hilfiker, R., Amit, O., Scheidhauer, A., Andrews, B.,..... Ettlin, T. (2011). Best practice for motor imagery: A systematic literature review on motor imagery training elements in five different disciplines. *BMC Medicine, 9,* 75.

Sharma, N., Simmons, L. H., Jones, P. S., Day, D. J., Carpenter, T. A., & Baron, J. (2009). Motor imagery after subcortical stroke: A functional magnetic resonance imaging study. *Stroke, 40*(4), 1315-1324.

Skoura, X., Personnier, P., Vinter, A., Pozzo, T., & Papaxanthis, C. (2008). Decline in motor prediction in elderly subjects: Right versus left arm differences in mentally simulated motor actions. *Cortex, 44*, 1271–1278.

Springer, A., Hamilton, A. F., & Cross, E. S. (2012). Simulating and predicting others' actions. *Psychological Research, 76*, 383-387.

Stinear, C. M., Byblow, W. D., Steyvers, M., Levin, O., & Swinnen, S. P. (2006). Kinesthetic, but not visual imagery modulates corticomotor excitability. *Experimental Brain Research, 168, 157-164.*

Suddendorf, T., & Moore, C. (2011). Introduction to the special edition: The development of episodic foresight. *Cognition Development, 26*, 295-298.

Voisin, J. I. A., Mercier, C., Jackson, P. L., Richards, C. L., & Malouin, F. (2011). Is Somatosensory excitiability more affected by the perspective or modality content of motor imagery? *Neuroscience Letters, 493*(1-2), 33-37.

Wintermute, S. (2012). Imagery in cognitive architecture: Representation and control at multiple evels of abstraction. *Cognitive Systems Research, 19-20*, 1-29.

Wohldmann, E. L., Healy, A. F., & Bourne, L. E. (2008) A mental practice superiority effect: Less retroactive interference and more transfer than physical practice. *Journal of Experimental Psychology: Learning, Memory, and Cognition, 34*(4), 823-833.

Wolpert, D. M. (1997). Computational approaches to motor control. *Trends in Cognitive Sciences, 1*, 209-216.

Young, S. J., Pratt, J, & Chau. T. (2009). Misperceiving the speed-accuracy tradeoff: Imagined Movements and perceptual decisions. *Experimental Brain Research, 192*(1), 121-132.

Zapparoli, L., Invernizzi, P., Gandola, M., Verardi, M., Berlingeri, M, Sherna, M.,…Paulesu, E. (2013). Mental images across the adult lifespan: a behavioural and fMRI investigation of motor execution and motor imagery. *Experimental Brain Research, 224*(4), 519-540.

Zhang, H., Xu, L., Wang, S., Xie, B., Gui, J., Long, Z., & Yao, L. (2011). Behavioral improvements and brain functional alterations by motor imagery training. *Brain Research, 1407,* 38-46.

Zuccaro, S. M., Steindler, R., Scena, S., & Costarella, M. (2012). Changes of psychical and physical conditions in the elderly after a four-year follow-up. *Archives of Gerontology and Geriatrics, 54,* 72-77.

In: Motor Imagery
Editor: Brandon M. Garcia

ISBN: 978-1-63483-125-3

Chapter 4

Motor Imagery with Brain-Computer Interface Neurotechnology

Christoph Guger[1], **Christoph Kapeller**[1], **Rupert Ortner**[1] and **Kyousuke Kamada**[2]*

[1]g.tec medical engineering GmbH, Guger Technologies OG, g.tec medical engineering Spain SL, g.tec neurotechnology USA Inc., Sierningstrasse, Schiedlberg.

[2]Department of Neurosurgery, School of Medicine, Asahikawa Medical University, Hokkaido, Japan

Abstract

A brain-computer interface (BCI) analyzes brain activity in real-time to convey information or control an external device. BCI systems often consist of a biosignal amplifier for EEG data acquisition, parameter estimation, and classification to make decisions in real-time. Many BCIs are controlled via motor imagery (through imagined movements), which modulates the EEG in certain frequency bands and regions. Motor imagery based BCIs are used for various applications like cursor control,

* guger@gtec.at

robotic and avatar control, stroke rehabilitation, cognitive assessment, training, and communication.

This article presents key scientific experiments and applications, including some of the newest results.

Keywords: Brain-computer interface, BCI, motor imagery, event-related desynchronization, ERD, rehabilitation, assessment, control applications

Introduction

What Is a BCI?

Brain-computer interfaces typically use the Electroencephalogram (EEG) or the Electrocorticogram (ECoG) to generate a control signal in real-time. Figure 1 illustrates the basic components of such a system. EEG based systems can easily be used with healthy subjects or patients, since the EEG is measured with active surface electrodes placed on the head, which may be dry electrodes or require electrode gel, saltwater, or other materials to ensure a good contact with the scalp. ECoG based BCI systems are mostly used with patients undergoing brain surgery or invasive brain mapping, which use implantable electrode grids or strips that usually have 64 to 256 channels.

The EEG/ECoG electrodes are connected to a biosignal amplifier to magnify the signals, which are transmitted to a computer for real-time analysis. This processing system performs parameter extraction algorithms such as: (i) bandpower estimation; (ii) calculation of adaptive autoregressive parameters; (iii) variance estimation; and many other techniques. Afterwards, these calculated parameters are classified with classification algorithms like (i) linear discriminant analysis (LDA) or (ii) support vector machines (SVM). Finally, these algorithms produce an output which allows control of an external device in real-time. This control could entail spelling, moving a cursor on a monitor, or using a robotic device. Critically, the BCI user must be able observe the object being controlled. This provides feedback reflecting whether the intended task was executed successfully. Different publications have shown that this feedback loop helps to improve the accuracy and speed of a BCI system (Guger et al., 2001, 2003, 2012a; Neuper and Allison, 2014).

BCI Principles and Applications

BCI systems could use: (i) evoked potentials like the P300 or N200; (ii) steady-state evoked potentials (SSEPs); (iii) motor imagery; and/or (iv) slow waves. Slow wave based systems use just a few channels and require substantial training. They are inaccurate, allow very limited bandwidth, and are highly vulnerable to noise. Steady-state based systems often use visual stimuli with specific frequencies to generate brain activity at corresponding frequencies when users view them.

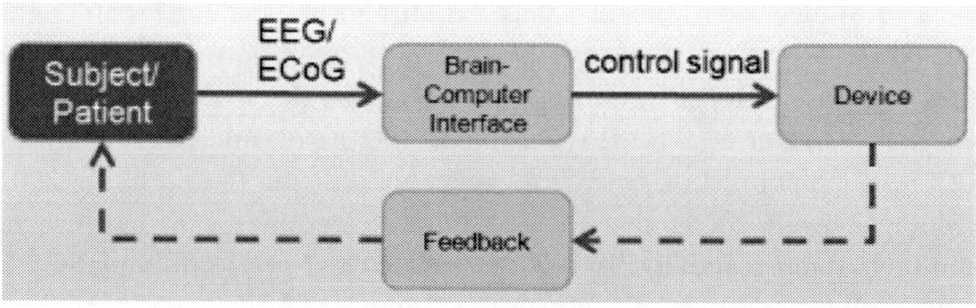

Figure 1. A brain-computer interface measures the EEG or ECoG from a healthy subject or patient, then uses signal processing algorithms to transform the signal into a control signal to operate an external device. The feedback loop is a key component that allows the user to see what s/he communicating or controlling, which allows higher accuracies.

These systems primarily use electrodes over the visual cortex, and can yield high accuracies with minimal training (Guger et al., 2012a). Speed and accuracy can be further improved if, instead of a constant stimulation frequency, a certain code is embedded in the stimulation by switching an LED on or off in a specific pattern. This code-based VEP or c-VEP approach has another advantage over SSVEP: c-VEP can be used with epilepsy patients without inducing seizures (Kapeller et al., 2014). SSVEP/cVEP based systems are perfectly suited for continuous control of external devices. BCIs with evoked potentials often use an oddball paradigm, in which an unlikely event is embedded in likely events, producing a P300 and other components in the EEG. P300 based systems also require very limited training time, with high accuracy and robustness (Guger et al., 2012b). P300 based system are used for goal-oriented control applications like smart home control, spelling, painting, and some online tasks (Edlinger et al., 2011).

Motor Imagery BCI Applications, Including Accuracy and Performance

Motor imagery based systems usually entail the imagination of right hand, left hand or foot movement. This produces an event-related desynchronization/synchronization (ERD/ERS) over the sensorimotor cortex, which the BCI can analyze to infer user intent. Therefore, the electrodes are placed over sensorimotor regions, and people are trained with feedback paradigms to gain control. In the case of EEG based systems, the BCI system uses either bipolar derivations over the motor cortex (Guger et al., 2001) or a whole grid of electrodes over the sensorimotor cortex analyzed with common spatial patterns or CSP (Guger et al., 1999). Ortner showed that the grand average accuracy after 20 minutes of training for the CSP based system is around 80% (Ortner et al., 2015, accepted). If 2 bipolar derivations are used, about 6% of the population reach 90% accuracy or better (Guger et al., 2003).

Motor imagery BCIs that include ECoG electrodes can also use task-related high-gamma activity. In this case, the ECoG grids are implanted over the sensorimotor cortex by a neurosurgeon. Standard grids have (for example) 64 electrode contacts with a center-to-center distance of 1 cm. High-density grids have 256 channels with a center-to-center distance of only a few mm, yielding a higher resolution. The first task for an ECoG based BCI system is the identification of the electrodes coding the necessary information. This can be done with a high-gamma functional mapping system within a few minutes (Brunner et al., 2009, Prückl et al., 2013; Kapeller et al., 2015, Schalk et al., 2008). Another approach is to train a spatial filter (CSP) to automatically weight each electrode according to the BCI classification task. This spatially filtered signal, or the selected electrode, can be used to directly control motor movements of a virtual or robotic avatar.

Advantages of Motor Imagery BCIs for these Applications

Motor imagery BCIs require more training time than P300 or SSVEP based systems, but can also yield high accuracies. They can be used for continuous control applications or detection of motor movements. This article will detail three applications: (i) motor rehabilitation after stroke; (ii) assessment of patients with disorders of consciousness; and (iii) avatar control to increase embodiment with (for example) a robotic avatar. For motor rehabilitation, the system can detect motor commands from the brain in real-time, which can be used to trigger a functional electrical stimulator (FES) or an avatar immediately after the movement imagery. This approach guarantees a close relationship between the movement imagery and other system activities (Daly, 2013, Mrachacz-Kersting, 2013, Thompson, 2013).

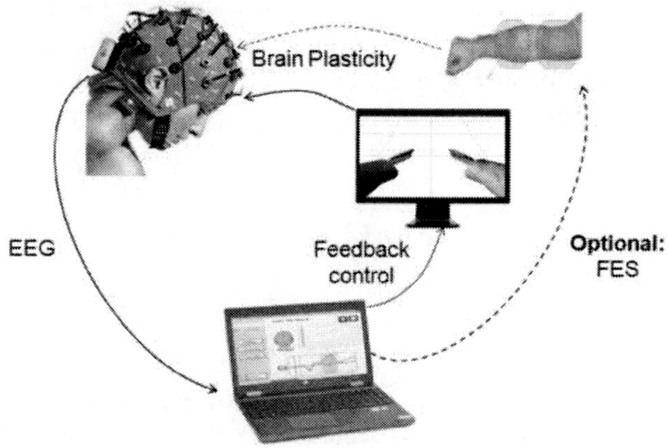

Figure 2. System components of a BCI system for rehabilitation.

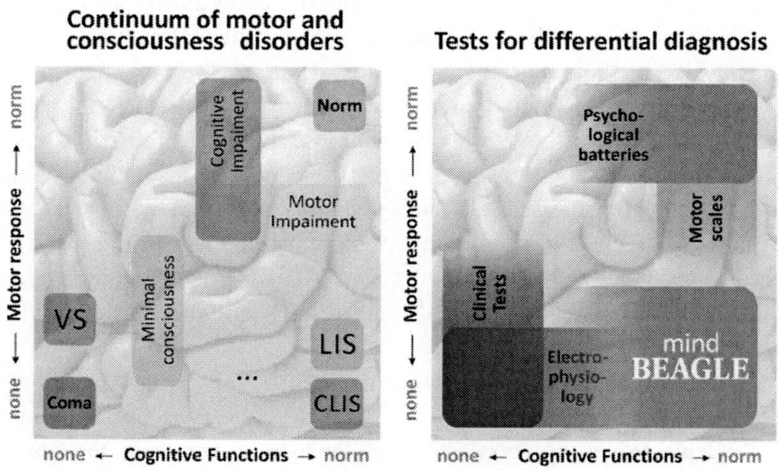

Figure 3. Left: Overview of motor and cognitive functions for different patients. Patients near the bottom of this figure have limited or no motor control, and may be unable to communicate (or even participate in assessments) without a BCI. Right: Electrophysiological test battery for assessment of cognitive functions for patients without adequate motor control.

For assessment purposes, the patient with DOC (see Figure 3) can be instructed to repeatedly imagine a certain motor movement. The BCI system calculates a certain classification accuracy that reflects the patients' cognitive processing capability (Guger, C. et al., 2014, Kotchoubey, B. et al., 2005, Kübler, A. et al., 2007, Laureys, S. et al., 2010).

Avatar control can be realized by directly mapping motor imagination onto real motor actions of a robotic avatar or a virtual representation. Motor imagery based BCIs guarantee a high embodiment with the artificial avatar. An important aspect for such applications is also the restoration of sensation of the prosthetic limb (Pisotta et al., 2014).

Methods

EEG/ECoG Recording Setups

Figure 4 shows the principal setup of a fully equipped EEG based BCI research lab. Normally, a person is seated in a comfortable chair with a head-rest to reduce artifacts. The person wears an electrode cap with 8-256 EEG electrodes, depending on the application, connected to the biosignal amplifier. Wireless technology allows the person to move around during the experiment or during breaks. The biosignal amplifier sends the data to the real-time processing BCI system that controls either: (i) a head-mounted display for stereoscopic effects; (ii) a computer monitor; or (iii) a Virtual Reality system to provide feedback to the user. Electrical stimulation, tactile stimulation or auditory stimulation can also be presented, and activity from microphones, eye-trackers and switches/buttons can be synchronized with the EEG data. The output of the BCI system can also be sent to a movement computer controlling an exoskeleton or a rehabilitation device. All of these components must communicate with each other in real-time to fully automate the experimental setup.

ECoG based BCI systems are typically used with patients who are seated in a bed in front of a computer screen or Virtual Reality system (see Figure 5). The ECoG electrodes are implanted by a neurosurgeon, and the electrode cables are connected to the 64-256 channel amplifier system. The data are transmitted to the BCI system, which has to deal with much more data because of the higher sampling frequency. This system can be synchronized with more or less the same components as the EEG system.

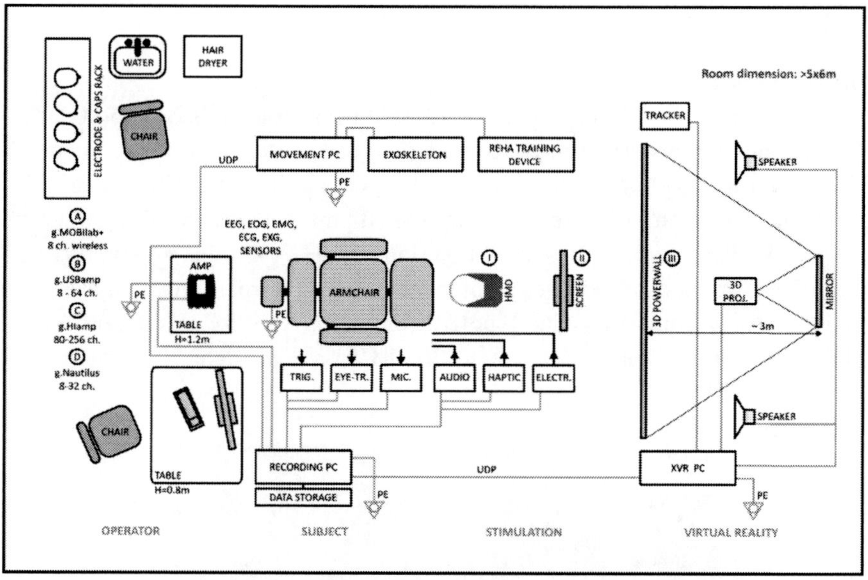

Figure 4. Laboratory plan of a complete EEG based brain-computer interface.

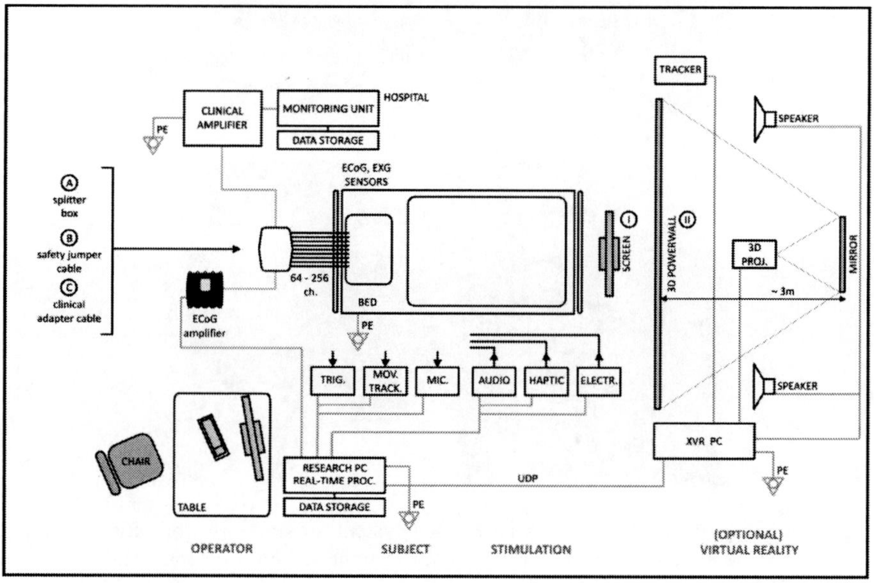

Figure 5. Laboratory plan of a complete ECoG based brain-computer interface.

System Setup for Each Application

Motor Rehabilitation with BCI

Figure 6 illustrates the experimental setup for motor rehabilitation with a 64 channel BCI system. The 64 channel cap uses active electrodes for quick EEG cap preparation and clean, artifact free data collection. These electrodes are connected to the biosignal amplifier g.HIamp (g.tec medical engineering GmbH, Austria) with 24 Bit resolution and 256 Hz sampling frequency. The amplifier is connected to the computer running all the real-time analyses. The patient is also equipped with bipolar stimulation electrodes on both arms, which can move the hands when the BCI system detects a movement imagination.

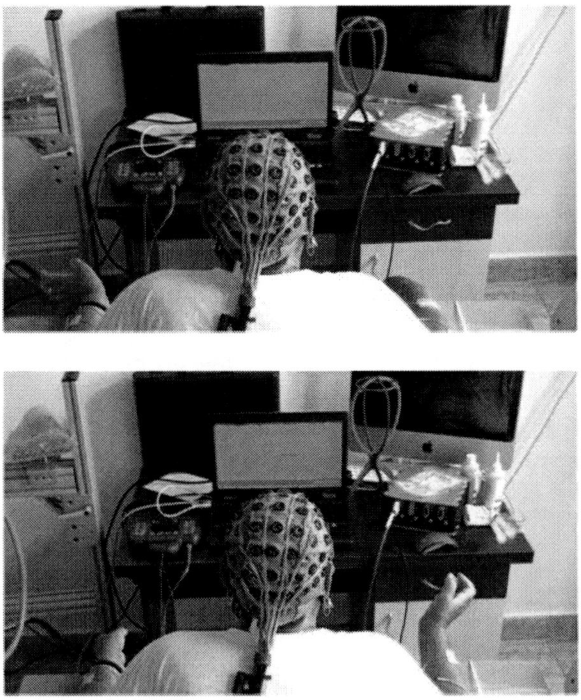

Figure 6. Setup of a motor imagery based BCI system for stroke rehabilitation with FES. Left: The patient imagines a left hand movement, which is detected and translated into a control signal with the BCI in real-time. This activates the FES and thereby moves the left hand. Right: Right hand movement imagination with right hand stimulation.

The system starts with an instruction arrow pointing either to the right or left side of the screen and by moving the avatar's hand (see Figure 7). This indicates the supposed motor movement imagination that the user should perform for 4 seconds. In total, the user has to imagine 80 left and 80 right hand movements, which requires about 25 minutes. During this procedure, the EEG data are acquired and the BCI system is calibrated. In the next run, the user can already control the avatar's arms or legs with the BCI's real-time output, thus creating closed-loop feedback.

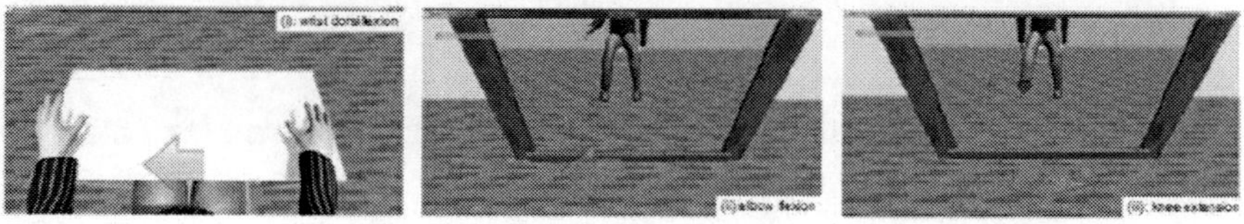

Figure 7. Experimental instructions are shown to the patient with right and left arrows indicating the site of hand movement imagination. The virtual hand moves if the BCI system detects the corresponding movement type. Left: Hand rehabilitation with first person view; Middle and Right: foot rehabilitation via a mirror to allow the patient to see his or her legs.

EEG DOC Assessment

To provide cognitive assessment for DOC patients, the user is prepared for recording with a cap with 16 EEG electrodes overlaying the sensorimotor cortex. Then, the user is instructed via the loudspeaker to imagine moving the left or right hand, and a short beep later indicates the termination of this movement imagination. This is repeated 60 times for each hand to keep the measurement time short. After an initial EEG acquisition run, the BCI system can be calibrated to give feedback in the next session. In this application, the feedback is for the experimenter and physician to investigate the success of motor control on the fly.

ECoG Avatar Control

In the case of ECoG based avatar control, the user is seated in front of the computer screen that cues which hand movement should be imagined (see Figure 8). The implant with 60 channels is connected to the BCI system, and the BCI controls an avatar's prosthetic hand in real-time, so that the user can directly see its movement. The tasks in this example were to imagine a fist, to make a peace sign or to straighten all fingers (each 20 times).

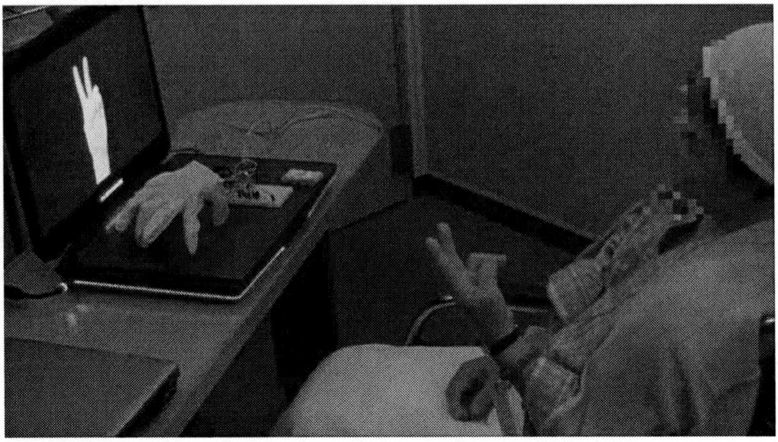

Figure 8. Epilepsy patient with ECoG implant connected to the BCI system. The patient is seated about 1 m in front of the computer screen that provides the instructions for certain motor movements. In this example, the monitor cues the patient to straighten all fingers. The robotic hand on the computer is controlled via the BCI output.

Signal Processing and Classification

In all three applications, the acquired EEG data from the first run are used to calculate a common-spatial pattern (CSP) filter. This filter has all EEG channels as inputs, and weights each channel according its importance for the discrimination task. It also maximizes the difference between the classification tasks. Then, the variance with a certain forgetting window is estimated for the most important filtered channels. These parameters are normalized, and finally a linear discriminant analysis is trained on the data. This results in a user-specific classifier that can be used to give feedback or to control an object in the next run.

Results

Motor Rehabilitation

Figure 9 shows both the mean and minimum classification error rates across 21 training sessions for one patient. The patient started with an error rate of 12.5% and improved to 3.8% after 13 sessions. The minimum error rate was never above 21.6%. Figure 9 (middle) also shows the 4 most important CSP filters for sessions 1 and 13. In both cases, the right and left finger regions (around C3 and C4) are the most important centers for the BCI classification.

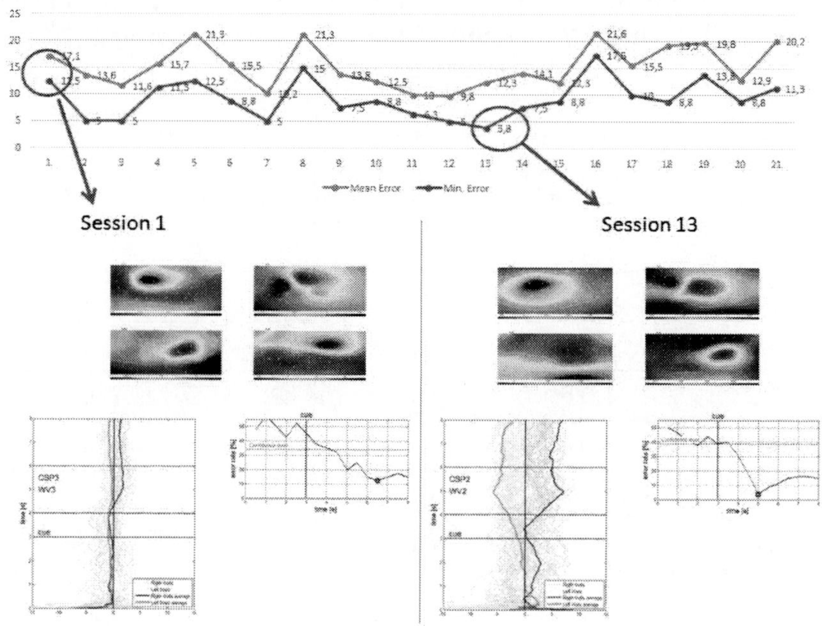

Figure 9. Classification accuracy, common spatial patterns (CSP) maps and cursor movement time for one subject, with classification accuracy over time. The mean error rate is calculated for the interval 2-4 seconds after the cue indicating the movement type. The minimum error rate is the minimum of the whole period after the cue (5 seconds).

The bottom line of Figure 9 shows the output of the LDA classifier for left and right movement imagery. In session 1, the difference between left and right hand imagery is much smaller than in session 13. Furthermore, the time course of the error rate over the movement imagination trials is shown. In session 13, the error drops more quickly and is ultimately lower than earlier sessions.

Table 1 summarizes performance in a 9-hole PEG test that the patient performed during the 21 BCI training sessions. This test of hand motor control requires users to put objects into holes, and the completion time and error rate is measured. The patient initially needed 31 seconds for the left (non-affected) hand, and 1 min 5 seconds for the right hand, which was affected by stroke. After the 21 BCI training sessions, the patient could complete the task within about 30 seconds for both hands.

Table 1. Results with a 9-hole PEG test, repeated 8 times for each hand. "Falls" reflects the number of times that a peg was dropped, reflecting an error

9-hole PEG test				
Date: 2014	Left hand	Falls	Right hand	Falls
24-06	31"	0	1'5''	0
26-06	32"	0	54"	0
29-06	32"	0	45"	0
2-07	31"	0	42"	0
6-09	31"	0	42"	0
9-09	29"	0	38"	0
12-09	29"	0	34"	0
15-09	29"	0	30"	0

Assessment of Cognitive Functions with Motor Imagery

Figure 10 presents the ERD/ERS maps for right and left hand movements over channels C3 and C4, and shows clear ERD and ERS activity. The bottom curve shows the classification accuracy over trial time for all movement imagination. The user reached a mean classification accuracy of 99.2%.

Avatar Control

Figure 11 shows a high density electrode grid with 60 channels implanted in an epilepsy patient at Asahikawa Medical University over the sensorimotor cortex. The other grid and strip electrodes are not used for the analysis presented here, since they are not located above the motor cortex.

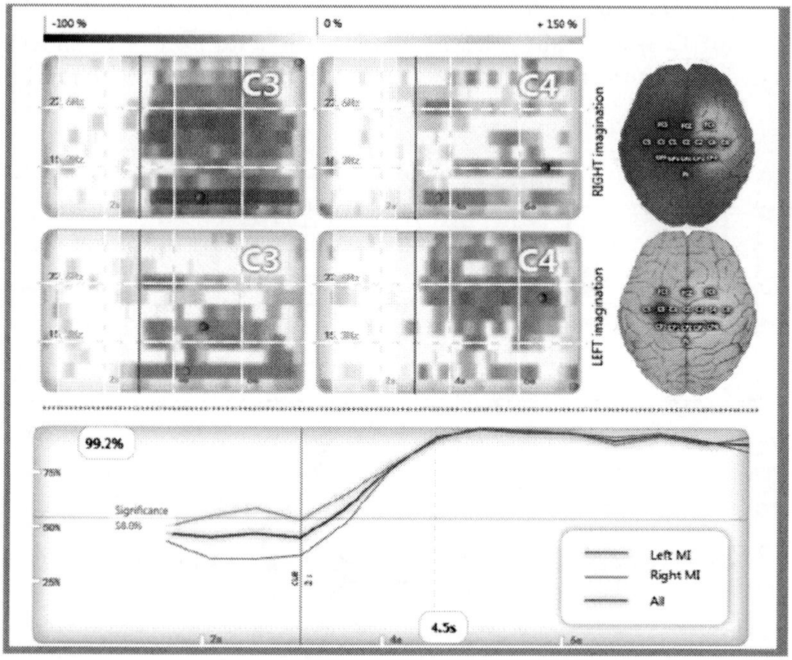

Figure 10. Top: ERD maps for electrode positions C3 and C4 for left and right hand movement imagination. Bottom: BCI classification accuracy over time.

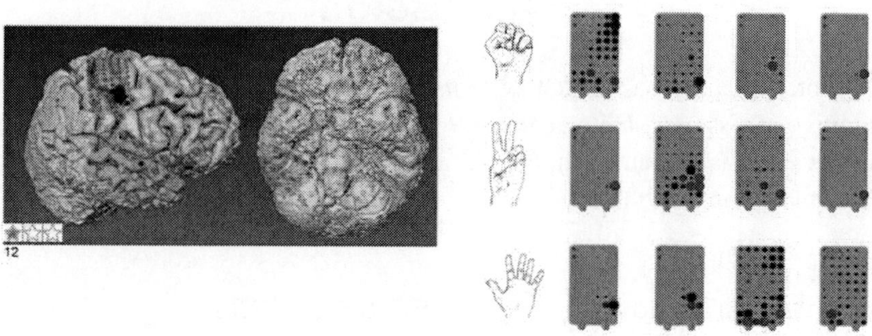

Figure 11. Brain mapping results from cortiQ indicating the ECoG electrodes responsible for motor movements. Left: ECoG grid locations superimposed on the brain. Right: CSP maps (fist, peace sign and fingers straight) on a high density grid for the 4 most important CSP filters.

Figure 11 (right) shows the 4 most important CSP filters for the three types of motor movement imaginations. The red and blue circles around the electrodes indicate important electrodes for a certain movement task (bigger diameter = more important).

Figure 12 shows the classification error rate over 120 movement repetitions across the trial duration. The patient reached a minimum error rate of 0%.

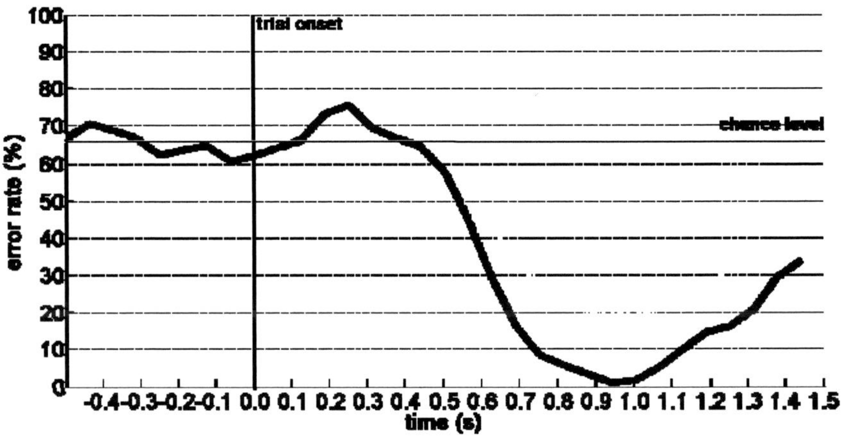

Figure 12. Classification error over time for one subject. The red line reflects stimulus onset, when the subject was first cued to perform left vs. right motor imagery.

Discussion

Motor imagery based BCI systems are important for motor rehabilitation, cognitive assessment and avatar control to increase embodiment. This chapter has reviewed relevant technology, and shown how it is used in certain experimental approaches.

Advantages/Disadvantages of EEG based BCIs

EEG based systems have the major advantages of being easy to prepare and use, without requiring the costs, risks, and other challenges associated with neurosurgery. New technologies such as active electrodes, 24 bit resolution and high oversampling to reduce noise have made these systems much easier in real-world applications. Within about two minutes, a user can be prepared for recording with a cap using 16 EEG channels, which can be adequate for motor rehab and cognitive assessment. Therefore, this procedure can easily be done on a regular basis. Another important advantage is that the active EEG electrodes can be mounted without abrading the skin, which makes the procedure much more comfortable for the patient and therapist. Additionally, water based gel don't cause skin irritation or itching, and the gel may disappear a few hours after the EEG cap is removed.

Advantages/Disadvantages of ECoG based BCIs

The implanted ECoG grids have the big advantage of high spatial resolution, which allows BCIs to discriminate individual finger movements, a task which is impossible with EEG based systems. Furthermore, the signal-to-noise ratio of an ECoG system is much higher, which makes it easier to capture a good control signal, quickly identify the important electrodes and establish reliable communication and control. Critically, the ECoG based BCI system does not produce many false positives, which allows the system to reliably stop the avatar or hand movement if the user is done with the control task. This "zero-class problem" is especially difficult with EEG based systems. However, the zero-class problem is not relevant for the two presented applications: (i) motor rehabilitation and (ii) cognitive assessment.

Advantages/Disadvantages of BCIs for assessment and rehabilitation

BCI systems for cognitive assessment have the major advantage of providing a very objective measure of each patient's task performance. If the BCI accuracy is 0%, then it is very likely that the patient cannot perform the task; if the accuracy is 100%, then the patient was able to perform the task very well. This informs the therapist whether the patient is still able to follow conversations and understand instructions.

In the case of motor rehabilitation, the BCI classification informs the therapist whether or not the patient is correctly performing the task. This allows the therapist to influence the training and motivate the patient. The paired stimulation with motor imagery also produces motor movement, which further motivates the patient to perform the training.

Future Outlook

In the future, a combination of these systems will be important. Motor rehabilitation systems will also be used for patients with DOC, while cognitive assessment systems will be used for patients with motor disabilities. The full body avatar could provide the perfect closed-loop feedback device in the future, and will open many new applications like self-feeding with your own avatar (Figure 13).

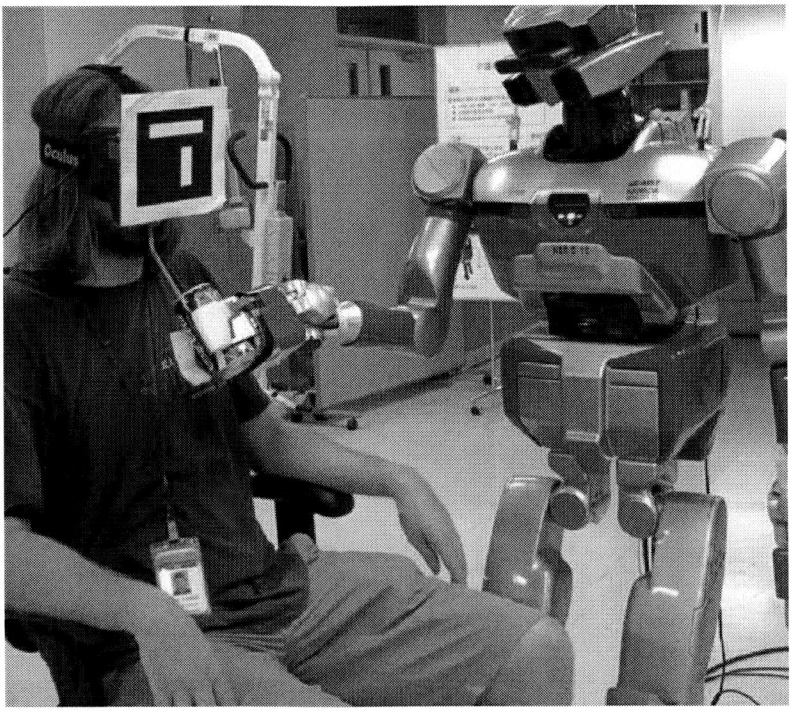

Figure 13. A BCI user controlling his avatar to give him a Coke from Abderrahmane Kheddar (CNRS-AIST JRL) (Petit et al., 2015).

References

Brunner, P., et al. (2009). A practical procedure for real-time functional mapping of eloquent cortex using electrocorticographic signals in humans. *Epilepsy & Behavior* 15.3, 278-286.

Daly, J.J. (2013). Brain-computer interface applied to motor recovery after brain injury, In: Introduction to neural engineering for motor rehabiliation, Eds: Farina, D., Jensen, W., Akay, M., IEEE Press Wiley, 463-476.

Edlinger, G., Hintermueller, C., & Guger, G. (2011). A hybrid BCI using P300 and SSVEP for smart home control. In: *Proceedings of the Neuroscience 2011.* November 12 – 16, 2011. Washington D.C., USA. p. 51.

Guger, C., Ramoser, H., Neuper, C., & Pfurtscheller, G. (1999). Rapid BCI Prototyping: Results with adaptive autoregressive parameters and common spatial patterns. In: *BCI Technology: Theory and Practice, First International Meeting,* Rensselaerville, USA.

Guger, C., Schlögl, A., Neuper, C., Walterspacher, D., Strein, T., & Pfurtscheller, G. (2001). Rapid prototyping of an EEG-based brain-computer interface (BCI). *IEEE Transactions on Neural Systems and Rehabilitation Engineering,* 9(1), 49-58.

Guger, C., Edlinger, G., Harkam, W., Niedermayer, I., & Pfurtscheller, G. (2003). How many people are able to operate an EEG-based brain-computer interface (BCI)? *IEEE Transactions on Neural Systems and Rehabilitation Engineering,* 11(2), 145-7.

Guger, C., Allison, B. Z., Großwindhager, B., Prückl, R., Hintermüller, C., Kapeller, C., Bruckner, M., Krausz, G., & Edlinger, G. (2012a). How Many People Could Use an SSVEP BCI? *Frontiers in Neuroscience,* 19,6:169.

Guger, C., Krausz, G., Allison, B. Z., & Edlinger, G. (2012b). Comparison of dry and gel based electrodes for P300 brain-computer interfaces. *Frontiers in Neuroscience,* 6, 60.

Guger, C., Sorger, B., Noirhomme, Q., Naci, L., Monti, M.M., Real, R., Pokorny, C., Veser, S., Lugo, Z., Quitadamo, L., Lesenfants, D., Risetti, M., Formisano, R., Toppi, J., Astolfi, L., Emmerling, T., Heine, L., Erlbeck, H., Horki, P., Kotchougey, B., Bianchi, L., Mattia, D., Goebel, R., Owen, A., Pellas, F., Laureys, S., Kübler, A., Cincotti, F. (2014). Brain-computer interfaces for assessment and communication in disorders of consciousness, In: Emerging Theory and Practice in Neuroprosthetics, Edt: Ganesh R. Naik, Yina Gui, *IGI Global,* 181-214.

Kapeller, C., Kamada, K., Ogawa, H., Prueckl, R., Scharinger, J., & Guger, C. (2014). An electrocorticographic BCI using code-based VEP for control in video applications: a single-subject study. *Front Syst. Neurosci.,* 7; 8:139.

Kapeller, C., Korostenskaja, M., Prueckl, R., Chen, P.C., Lee, K.H., Westerveld, M., Salinas, C.M., Cook, J.C., Baumgartner, J.E., & Guger, C. (2015). CortiQ-based Real-Time Functional Mapping for Epilepsy Surgery. *J. Clin. Neurophysiol. 2015* Feb 26. [Epub ahead of print].

Kapeller, C., Gergondet, P., Kamada, K., Ogawa, H., Takeuchi, F., Ortner, R., Prückl, R., Kheddar, A., Scharinger, J., Guger, C. (2015). Online control of a humanoid robot through hand movement imagination using CSP based ECoG features, EMBC, Milan, 2015, submitted.

Kotchoubey, B., Lang, S., Mezger, G., Schmalohr, D., Schneck, M., Semmler, A., et al. (2005). Information processing in severe disorders of consciousness: Vegetative state and minimally conscious state. Clinical Neurophysiology, 116(10), 2441-2453.

Kübler, A & Kotchoubey, B (2007). Brain-computer interfaces in the continuum of consciousness. Current Opinion in Neurology, 20, 643-649.

Laureys S, Celesia GG, Cohadon F, Lavrijsen J, León-Carrión J, Sannita WG, Sazbon L, Schmutzhard E, von Wild KR, Zeman A, Dolce G (2010). European Task Force on Disorders of Consciousness. Unresponsive wakefulness syndrome: a new name for the vegetative state or apallic syndrome. *BMC Med.* 1:8-68. doi: 10.1186/1741-7015-8-68.

Mrachacz-Kersting, N. (2013). Paired associative stimulation, In: Introduction to neural engineering for motor rehabiliation, Eds: Farina, D., Jensen, W., Akay, M., IEEE Press Wiley, 529-548.

Neuper, C. and Allison, B.Z. (2014). The B of BCIs: Neurofeedback principles and how they can yield clearer brain signals. In: Different psychological perspectives on cognitive processes: current research trends in Alps-Adria region, editors: Actis, R. and Galmonte, A., Cambridge University Press, 133-153.

Ortner, R., Scharinger, J., Lechner, A., & Guger, C. (2015). How many people can control a motor imagery based BCI using common spatial patterns? Neural Engineering (NER), 7th International IEEE/EMBS Conference, accepted for publication.

Pisotta, I, Ionta, S. (2014). Are we the robots? Man-machine integration, In: Emerging Theory and Practice in Neuroprosthetics, Edt: Ganesh R. Naik, Yina Gui, *IGI Global*, 81-100.

Damien Petit, Pierre Gergondet, Andrea Cherubini, Abderrahmane Kheddar, An integrated framework for humanoid embodiment with a BCI, *IEEE*

International Conference on Robotics and Automation (ICRA), May 26-30, 2015, Seattle, Washington.

Prueckl, R., Kapeller, C., Potes, C., Korostenskaja, M., Schalk, G., Lee, K.H., & Guger, C. (2013). CortiQ - clinical software for electrocorticographic real-time functional mapping of the eloquent cortex. *Conf. Proc. IEEE Eng. Med. Biol. Soc.* 2013; 2013:6365-8.

Schalk, G. , Leuthardt, E.C., Brunner, P., Ojemann, J.G., Gerhardt, L.A., Wolpaw, J.R. (2008). Real-time detection of event-related brain activity, *Neuroimage* 43 (2), 245–249.

Thompson, A.K., Wolpaw, J. (2013). Operant conditioning of spinal reflexes for motor rehabilitation after CNS damage, In: Introduction to neural engineering for motor rehabiliation, Eds: Farina, D., Jensen, W., Akay, M., IEEE Press Wiley, 549-570.

In: Motor Imagery
Editor: Brandon M. Garcia

ISBN: 978-1-63483-125-3

Chapter 5

Mental Practice: Neurophysiology and Clinical Aspects in Neurorehabilitation

Clarissa Cardoso dos Santos-Couto-Paz*
Faculty of Ceilândia, Universidade de Brasília (UnB),
Brasília, Distrito Federal, Brazil

Abstract

Motor imagery is an active cognitive strategy requiring the internal reproduction of a specific action without any overt motor output. Mental practice is a method by which the internal reproduction of a given motor act - the motor imagery - is extensively repeated. This method is defined as a mental rehearsal of kinesthetic and/or visual properties of movements. Actually, many studies showed that mental practice improves the functional performance in neurologic and orthopedic injuries associated with change in neural activation related to motor control. Usually this approach increases activation in motor areas related to planning and preparation and decreases activation in primary motor areas. This intervention can be used in physical therapy to improve motor

* Author's address and e-mail: Clarissa Cardoso dos Santos-Couto-Paz, Centro Metropolitano, conjunto A, lote 01, Brasília - DF. CEP: 72220-900, E-mail: clarissacardoso@unb.br, Telephone: +55 61 35430752

relearning in individuals with different motor impairments and physical functional disabilities. However, the definition of parameters is necessary to guide the application of this method in clinical practice. This chapter describes aspects related to the use of motor imagery in clinical practice, including: a) main indications in different injury stages, b) neurophysiologic aspects improving motor recovery in individuals with motor impairments, c) clinical parameters in physical therapy, including the assessment process, session's characteristics and follow-up, and d) clinical applicability. Many variables, such as the nature of motor tasks, practice intensity, duration, learning stages, as well as individual aspects, need to be considered to guide clinical practice. The knowledge of these variables helps to apply this approach in clinical contexts.

1. Motor Imagery and Mental Practice or Motor Imagery Practice

Motor imagery is a cognitive strategy that uses mental rehearsal or internal reproduction of a movement. Mental Practice (MP), or motor imagery practice, is a motor training method by which the motor imagery of a given motor act is extensively repeated with the intention of improving performance (Sharma, Baron, Rowe, 2009). Several studies, as well as physical therapy clinical practice, have shown the influence of mental practice in the increase of functional recovery in individuals with stroke, spinal cord injury, Parkinson's disease, and improvement of functional capacity in athletes.

Motor imagery may be divided into two perspectives or modalities: 1) first-person perspective or Kinesthetic Motor Imagery (KMI), or internal imagery, and 2) third-person perspective, Visual Motor Imagery (VMI) or external imagery. KMI involves imagining the feeling that the actual task performance produces, including the force and effort perceived during movement and balance (Callow and Waters, 2005), and VMI involves imagining seeing oneself performing the task. KMI produces significant modulation of the excitability in the primary motor cortex (M1), when compared to VMI (Stinear et al., 2005). Different studies have hinted at the importance of imagery perspective for sensorimotor reactivation in different motor impairments. Meugnot et al. (2015) suggested that KMI produces faster response in hand laterality tasks when compared with VMI in individuals with functional disability induced by brief period of limb nonuse. According to those authors, KMI may compensate the somatotopic effect of limb nonuse, and the slowdown of the sensorimotor processes, induced by 24 h of sensorimotor deprivation, may be counteracted by KMI, whereas no beneficial effect appeared with visual imagery.

Therefore, specific imagery modalities can serve different purposes. Previous research also demonstrated that directing the attention of athletes to the effects of their movements on the environment is more effective than focusing on the action itself. Previous studies showed that external visual imagery (EMI) can be more effective for form-based tasks, as athletes could easily visualize global positions and movements required for successful performance (Hardy and Callow, 1999; White and Hardy, 1995). However, internal visual imagery (IMI) would be better in goal-directed tasks (Callow et al., 2013; Callow and Roberts, 2012; White and Hardy, 1995).

2. Neurophysiology: The Motor Imagery-Based Mental Practice Is Similar to Motor Execution

Evidence indicates that motor deficits in cerebral injuries are related not only to problems with execution, but also to motor planning impairment. Motor imagery is the cognitive strategy that may be effective in helping motor planning. Previous studies suggested that motor imagery neurophysiological aspects are related to motor planning and preparation. Brain areas that are normally involved in movement planning and execution are also active during the imagination of a movement. Brain activation patterns, including temporal and special aspects during motor imagery, are similar to motor execution. During motor imagery, brain areas related to motor execution are activated. The areas activated during imagery, as well as during the execution of the movement, are the prefrontal cortex, pre-motor cortex, supplemental motor area, cingulate cortex, parietal cortex and cerebellum. However, the activation in the primary motor cortex is inconsistent (Vries and Mulder, 2007). According to Garrison, Winstein, Aziz-Zadeh (2010), motor imagery may rebuild planning and preparation areas rather than execution. The results of Kasses et al. (2009) showed the importance of the SMA not only for the preparation and execution of intended movements, but also for suppressing movements represented in the motor system but not performed, modeling M1 activation during motor imagery. In addition, during motor imagery and execution, similar variations occur in the autonomic nervous system (Thill et al., 1997). This variation can be used in clinical practice to control motor imagery during sessions (Santos-Couto-Paz et al., 2013).

3. Emerging Practices

Mental practice based on motor imagery has been used as motor training to improve functional capacity in a wide range of situations, including sports, recovery of motor activity after injury, neurodegenerative diseases and neuropathic pain.

3.1. Sports

Motor imagery can be effective in optimizing the execution of movements in athletes and this approach is better than no physical practice (Feltz and Landers, 1983; Driskell, Cooper, Moran, 1994). Recent studies have shown that different motor imagery perspectives could change different motor performances in sports. Yao el al. (2013) suggested that training by using internal motor imagery of forceful muscle contractions was effective in improving voluntary muscle strength without physical exercise. Results suggest that this training is likely to increase the cortical-spinal excitability that may have improved motor unit recruitment and activation, and led to greater muscle strength (Yao et al., 2013). Guilot et al. (2013) confirmed the effectiveness of external motor imagery, in addition to physical practice, to improve tennis serve performance (Guilot et al., 2013). Therefore, the choice of motor imagery perspective depends on the objective and motor task to be trained in sports.

3.2. Stroke

Individuals with chronic stroke increase functional performance with motor imagery practice. Probably, such individuals present motor impairment due to limitations in motor planning and preparation and not in motor execution. Mental practice may increase activation in brain areas related to motor planning and preparation in contralateral areas, and decrease activation in ipsilateral areas. Mental practice, in addition to task-specific practice therapy programs, increases affected arm use and is significantly more effective than task-specific practice alone, and can also change the activation of brain areas in chronic stroke patients presenting stable and moderate motor deficits (Page et al., 2009). Such patients received 30-minute therapy sessions for their affected arms and 30-minute mental practice sessions, occurring 3 days/week for 10 weeks, emphasizing important activities of daily living. According to Liu et al., (2004) and Santos-Couto-Paz et al., (2013), mental practice promotes relearning for people after a stroke. Interventions based on motor imagery showed better relearning of motor tasks and demonstrated greater ability to retain trained tasks after 1 month and to transfer relearned skills to other untrained tasks (Liu et al., 2004). In first study, inpatients, after a cerebral infarction, received 15 sessions (1h/day for 3 weeks) of either a mental imagery program or a conventional functional training intervention for the relearning of daily living tasks (Liu et al., 2004). Santos-Couto-paz et al. (2013) proposed a specific functional task-oriented mental practice in association with conventional physical therapy. According to that study, such approach led to improvements in motor imagery abilities combined with increases in the amount of use and quality of movement in daily functions, manual dexterity, and gait speed (Santos-Couto-Paz et al., 2013). Individuals with stable mild and moderate upper limb impairments participated of this study and one-on-one 30-minute mental practice training sessions during three days per week for four weeks, totaling 12 sessions. This training program was based on tasks selected according to the individuals' objectives with gradual increases in the task constraints related to the number of the kinematic aspects.

The studies were carried out on individuals with chronic stroke and stability of motor impairment. The results for acute stroke are inconclusive.

3.3. Parkinson' Disease

Few studies involving metal practice and Parkinson's disease appear in the literature. Therefore, since motor impairment in this population is related to supplemental motor area activity, such intervention can be used. Reduced activity in this region may be related to locomotor dysfunction (Peterson et al., 2014). Those authors showed that altered supplemental motor area activity in Parkinson's disease during imagined turning may represent compensatory neural adaptations during complex gait. Tamir, Dickstein and Huberman (2007) demonstrated that, especially for reducing bradykinesia, the combination of motor imagery and real practice may be effective in the treatment of Parkinson's disease. In this study, twelve patients with idiopathic Parkinson's disease received combined therapy, whereas 11 received physical therapy alone, during 1-h sessions, 2 times per week for 12 weeks. Comparable motor tasks provided to both groups included callisthenic exercises, functional tasks, and relaxation exercises. Therefore, probably, the mental practice program may be used to increase supplemental motor area activity and to improve the functional capacity in Parkinson's disease.

3.4. Spinal Cord Injury

Few studies have approached the relation between motor imagery and spinal cord injury. Further studies might probably confirm the potential role of mental practice in motor recovery within a larger sample. Two case studies showed the influence of mental practice and motor recovery in spinal cord injury (Grangeon et al., 2010; Grangeon et al., 2012). Those studies showed the influence of mental practice in improving upper limb rehabilitation, considering the functional prognostic after the spinal injury.

3.5. Brain Machine Interface

Motor imagery may be used to drive the brain-computer interface in strokes (Wang et al., 2010; Ang et al., 2008 and 2009) and spinal cord injury (Rohm et al., 2013). The use of motor imagery for brain-computer interface improves cortical changes associated to functional performance, thus helping gait and upper limb function robotic devices.

3.6. Pain

Changes in cortical processing and organization, considering the changes in sensorial and motor cortical areas, associated with perceptual disturbances, as well as poor responses to conventional treatments, characterize the phantom limb and complex regional pain syndrome. Considering neurophysiology mechanisms, mental practice can probably be used in phantom limb and complex regional pain syndrome. According to Moseley (2006), graded motor imagery is effective for a small subset of patients with type I complex regional pain syndrome. Motor imagery reduced pain and disability in such patients

(Moseley, 2004) or phantom limb pain (Moseley, 2006), but the mechanism, or mechanisms, of the effect are not clear.

Motor imagery can be used to reduce phantom member pain. Beaumont et al. (2011), in a single-case multiple baseline study, included six persons with upper or lower phantom limb pain, and suggested that combining observation and imagination of movements can reduce phantom limb pain.

According to Moseley (2004), type I complex regional pain syndrome involves cortical abnormalities similar to those observed in phantom pain and after strokes. Therefore, possible explanations relating the influence of mental practice to neuropathic pain are the change in planning and preparation brain areas modulating somatosensory areas, or sustained and focused attention on the affected limb, or both. However, few studies have been developed for these specific conditions and neurophysiologic mechanisms (Dier et al., 2010). Additional studies are necessary to confirm the findings, elucidate the mechanisms and identify patients likely to respond.

4. Role in Physical Therapy

Mental practice is an inexpensive, low-cost method of intervention, but not an easy one. For clinical application in physical therapy one needs to understand the neurophysiological aspects related to the method and to know all factors related to the clinical use the method. Although the literature describes the increase in motor performance in different cases, including stroke, Parkinson's disease, spinal cord, neuropathic pain, and sports, the clinical aspects related to the application are not clearly described.

Many variables, such as the type of motor tasks trained, practice intensity, duration, learning stages and individual aspects, need to be considered to guide clinical practice. The knowledge of such variables can help this approach in clinical contexts.

Motor imagery must be understood as a cognitive strategy that can be used when motor impairment is related to motor planning and preparation. Therefore, the physical therapist needs to know the neurophysiological aspects related to mental practice to choose the best parameters for a specific motor impairment.

Therefore, in order to perform mental practice in physical therapy clinical practice, one needs to consider various aspects, including: a quiet environment, 30- to 60-minute sessions, and a number of sessions defined according to the intervention objective. In addition, individual sessions lead to better results. Environment factors, including pictures and videos related to the movements and tasks trained, can be used to guide the motor imagery. Some studies (Page et al., 2009; Liu et al., 2004) used pictures and videos during mental practice. Santos-Couto-Paz et al., (2013) used environment strategies based in the task's kinematic characteristics in the motor imagery. This factor can influence the motor imagery perspective and consequently the cortical changes and motor recovery. Another aspect related to the intervention session is the motor imagery perspective. Probably, the choice of the motor imagery perspective is related to the treatment objective. For example, in sports, the visual motor imagery is frequently used, while in neuro-rehabilitation the kinesthetic motor imagery is more used, due to the increase in the activation in motor and proprioceptive areas.

The choice of the task to be trained must be based on the initial assessments and individual objectives. Previous studies reported that functional task-oriented motor training showed a higher increase in motor performance than training based on isolated movements; it is possible that mental practice based on functional tasks can produce a better learning (Santos-Couto-Paz et al., 2013; Santos-Couto-Paz et al., 2015).

Before starting the sessions, it is necessary to identify the motor imagery skills. Several instruments have been used to assess such skills. The individual needs to present the ability to adequately perform the motor imagery. Individuals with motor apraxia can present difficulty with the imagery. Greg, Hall, Martin (2007) suggested that a revised motor imagery questionnaire (MIQ-RS) is an appropriate instrument for the assessment of visual and kinesthetic movement imagery skills. The Kinesthetic and Visual Imagery Questionnaire (KVIQ) presents adequate psychometric properties that support their use in healthy individuals and post-stroke persons (Malouin et al., 2007).

In addition, assessing motor performance is important when defining the treatment objective. Motor skills must be assessed, and the following tests were used: (1) Minnesota Manual Dexterity Test and Motor Activity Log (Santos-Couto-Paz et al., 2013), Action Research Arm Test and the upper extremity section of the Fugl-Meyer Assessment (Page et al., 2007; Page et al., 2009) for upper limb functions; (2) 7-point Likert scale for patient's competence level in performing both trained and untrained tasks; (3) Color Trails Test (Liu et al., 2004) for motor learning assessment; (4) clinical instruments such as 10-m walk test (Oostra et al., 2015, Santos-Couto-Paz et al., 2013) and Timed "Up & Go" Test for gait assessment; (4) Tinetti Balance and Gait Evaluation Scale (Beauches et al., 2015, Zangrando et al., 2015) for balance assessment.

Therefore, in order to assess motor disabilities and motor imagery skills, it is important to identify whether motor imagery is an adequate therapeutic strategy to improve motor performance and to measure the gain in functional performance after the program. For that purpose, it is necessary to know the psychometric proprieties of such instruments and their clinical applications.

5. Clinical Implications

Motor imagery practice, or mental practice, is considered a therapeutic strategy to increase motor performance in individuals with chronic and sub-acute motor impairment related to motor planning and preparation. Previous definition of the parameters is important to perform motor imagery in clinical practice. Therefore, the selection of the assessment instrument, the aspects related to clinical execution, including the environment, professional expertise, motor imagery modalities, the selection of movements or tasks trained based on the main complaints and repetitions and number of sessions are essential for the appropriate application of this method in clinical contexts.

References

Beauchet O, Launay CP, Fantino B, Annweiler C, Allali G. Motor imagery of gait in non-demented older community-dwellers: performance depends on serum 25-hydroxyvitamin D concentrations. *Age* (Dordr). 2015 Apr;37(2):18.

Beaumont G, Mercier C, Michon PE, Malouin F, Jackson PL. Decreasing phantom limb pain through observation of action and imagery: a case series. *Pain Med.* 2011 Feb;12(2):289-99.

Callow N, Roberts R, Hardy L, Jiang D, Edwards MG. Performance improvements from imagery: evidence that internal visual imagery is superior to external visual imagery for slalom performance. *Frontiers in Human Neuroscience* 2013; 7: Article 697.

Callow N, Roberts R. Visual imagery perspectives and preference: conceptualization and measurement. *J. Ment. Image.* 2012: 36:31–39.

Callow N, Waters A. The effect of kinesthetic imagery on the sport confidence of flat-race jockeys. *Psychology of Sport and Exercise* 2005; 6: 443-459.

Diers M, Christmann C, Koeppe C, Ruf M, Flor H. Mirrored, imagined and executed movements differentially activate sensorimotor cortex in amputees with and without phantom limb pain. *Pain.* 2010 May;149(2):296-304.

Driskell JE, Copper C, Moran A. Does mental practice enhance performance? *J. Sport Psychol* 1994; 79: 481–492.

Feltz DL, Landers DM. The effects of mental practice on motor skill learning and performance: a meta-analysis. *J. Sport Psychol* 1983; 5: 25–57.

Garrison KA, Winstein CJ, Aziz-Zadeh L. The Mirror Neuron System: A Neural Substrate for Methods in Stroke Rehabilitation. *Neurorehabil Neural Repair.* 2010; 5: 1-9.

Grangeon M, Guillot A, Sancho PO, Picot M, Revol P, Rode G, Collet C. Rehabilitation of the elbow extension with motor imagery in a patient with quadriplegia after tendon transfer. *Arch. Phys. Med. Rehabil.* 2010; Jul;91 (7):1143-6.

Grangeon M, Revol P, Guillot A, Rode G, Collet C. Could motor imagery be effective in upper limb rehabilitation of individuals with spinal cord injury? A case study. *Spinal Cord.* 2012; Oct;50(10):766-71.

Gregg M, Hall C, Butler A. The MIQ-RS: A Suitable Option for Examining Movement Imagery Ability. eCAM Advance Access 2007.

Guillot A, Desliens S, Rouyer C, Rogowski I. Motor imagery and tennis serve performance: the external focus efficacy. *J. Sports Sci. Med.* 2013; Jun 1;12(2):332-8. eCollection 2013.

Hardy L, Callow N. Efficacy of external and internal visual imagery perspectives for the enhancement of performance on tasks in which form is important. *J. Sport Exerc. Psychol.* 1999; 21: 95–112.

Kasess CH, Windischberger C, Cunnington R, Lanzenberger R, Pezawas L, Moser E. The suppressive inflence of SMA on M1 in motor imagery revealed by fMRI and dynamic causal modeling. *NeuroImage.*2008; Apr;40(2):828-37.

Liu KP, Chan CC, Lee TM, Hui-Chan CW. Mental imagery for promoting relearning for people after stroke: a randomized controlled trial. *Arch. Phys. Med. Rehabil.* 2004; Sep;85(9):1403-8.

Malouin F, Richards C, Jackson PL, Lafleur MF, Durand A, Doyon J. The Kinesthetic and Visual Imagery Questionnaire (KVIQ) for Assessing Motor Imagery in Persons with Physical Disabilities: A Reliability and

Construct Validity Study. *Journal of Neurologic Physical Therapy*: 2007 Mar:31(1): 20-29

Meugnot A, Agbangla NF, Almecija Y, Toussaint L. Motor imagery practice may compensate for the slowdown of sensorimotor processes induced by short-term upper-limb immobilization. *Psychol. Res.* 2015 May;79(3):489-99.

Moseley GL. Graded motor imagery for pathologic pain: a randomized controlled trial. *Neurology*. 2006; Dec 26;67(12):2129-34. Epub 2006 Nov 2.

Moseley GL. Graded motor imagery is effective for long-standing complex regional pain syndrome: a randomised controlled trial. *Pain*. 2004 Mar;108(1-2):192-8.

Oostra KM, Oomen A, Vanderstraeten G, Vingerhoets G. Influence of motor imagery training on gait rehabilitation in sub-acute stroke: A randomized controlled trial. *J. Rehabil Med.* 2015 Feb 23;47(3):204-9.

Page SJ, Levine P, Khoury JC. Modified constraint-induced therapy combined with mental practice: Thinking through better motor outcomes. *Stroke.* 2009; 40:551-4.

Peterson DS, Pickett KA, Duncan RP, Perlmutter JS, Earhart GM. Brain activity during complex imagined gait tasks in Parkinson disease. *Clin. Neurophysiol.* 2014; May;125 (5):995-1005.

Rohm M1, Schneiders M, Müller C, Kreilinger A, Kaiser V, Müller-Putz GR, Rupp R. Hybrid brain-computer interfaces and hybrid neuroprostheses for restoration of upper limb functions in individuals with high-level spinal cord injury. *Artif. Intell Med.* 2013; Oct;59(2):133-42.

Santos-Couto-Paz CC, Salmela LFT, Tierra-Criollo CJ. The addition of functional task-oriented mental practice to conventional physical therapy improves motor skills in daily functions after stroke. *Braz J. Phys. Ther.* 2013; Nov-Dec; 17(6):564-71.

Santos-Couto-Paz CC, Salmela LFT, Tierra-Criollo CJ, Martins EF. Imagética motora em pacientes pós-acidente vascular encefálico. In: Associação Brasileira de Fisioterapia Neurofuncional; Garcia CSNB, Facchinetti LD, organizadoras. PROFISIO Programa de Atualização em Fisioterapia Neurofuncional: Ciclo 2. Porto Alegre: *Artmed Panamericana;* 2015 p. 9-36. (Sistema de Educação Continuada a Distância, v.2).

Sharma N, Baron JC, Rowe JB. Motor imagery after stroke: Relating outcome to motor network connectivity. *Ann. Neurol.* 2009;66:604-16.

Stinear CM, Byblow WD, Steyvers M, Levin O, Swinnen SP. Kinesthetic, but not visual, motor imagery modulates corticomotor excitability. *Exp. Brain Res.* 2006; 168:157- 64.

Tamir R, Dickstein R, Huberman M. Integration of motor imagery and physical practice in group treatment applied to subjects with Parkinson's disease. *Neurorehabil Neural Repair.* 2007; Jan-Feb;21(1):68-75.

Thill EE, Bryche D, Poumarat G, Rigoulet N. Task-involvement and ego-involvement goals during actual and imagined movements: their effects on cognitions and vegetative responses. *Behavioural Brain Research.* 1997, 82:159-67.

Vries S, Mulder T. Motor imagery and stroke rehabilitation: a critical discussion. *J. Rehabil Med* 2007; 39: 5–13.

White A, Hardy L. Use of different imagery perspectives on the learning and performance of different motor skills. *Br. J. Psychol.* 1995; 86: 169–180.

Yao WX, Ranganathan VK, Allexandre D, Siemionow V, Yue GH. Kinesthetic imagery training of forceful muscle contractions increases brain signal and muscle strength. *Front Hum. Neurosci.* 2013; Sep 26;7:561.

Zangrando F, Piccinini G, Pelliccioni A, Saraceni VM, Paolucci T. Neurocognitive rehabilitation in Parkinson's disease with motor imagery: a rehabilitative experience in a case report. *Case Rep. Med.* 2015: Article ID 670385, 4 pages.

Index

A

B

C

F

G

H

I

J

T

U

V

W

Y